TESTAMENTS OF TRANSFORMATION
EVOLVE EMERGE EXPAND: Return to Your Authentic Self

'It's a simple concept... but how do we actually put it into practice? Jennifer Kupcho's *Evolve, Emerge, Expand: Return to Your Authentic Self* serves as a roadmap to self-love—and it's a roadmap with choices. In this book, Jennifer invites you to unweave the tapestry of your life, gently pulling out the threads of your past to uncover your authentic truth. By exploring these layered experiences, you can create pathways to emerge from doubt. Jennifer's inspiring and liberating message guides you toward expansion through positivity, not conformity.

Her insights, shared with warmth and understanding, are drawn from her own life experiences. I found myself relating to her journey and recognizing parallels in mine. Life, as Jennifer so beautifully illustrates, is not linear but circuitous. This accessible, reader-friendly guide personalizes your journey and offers choices—just as life does. Gather your tribe and discover your true, Authentic Self."
~SUSAN KRATOCHVIL

'Reading *Evolve, Emerge, Expand: Return to Your Authentic Self* brings both joy and tears. As a people pleaser throughout my entire life, I thought that was normal. I was pleasing everyone but myself. The stories Jennifer shares along with the tools to work with are beautiful. I finally don't feel alone. Everything written is so relatable and I can't wait for women everywhere to feel the same experience. Through this book I am now learning to become my Authentic Self. I'm listening to my instincts and finding my voice step by step. Thank you, Jennifer, from the bottom of my heart.'
~PATRICIA AMORE

'Jennifer Kupcho's highly inspirational book resonates with those who wish to embark on their truest and greatest journeys moving forward. A powerful read for the heart, the soul, and the mind!'
~EDIE RINALDI

'The road to personal growth and fulfillment is always yours to choose. Whether you take the road less traveled or the path of least resistance, the journey is uniquely yours. In *Evolve, Emerge, Expand: Return to Your Authentic Self*, Jennifer offers a guiding light, making it easier for you to find the road that resonates with where you are in your process, ensuring a smoother and more aligned journey. This book is a beautiful gift—like having a life purpose coach in your back pocket, always within reach whenever you need guidance most.

Jennifer's "Path to Progress" progression is the cornerstone of this transformative guide. By following her carefully designed steps, you are assured of success, moving forward with confidence and clarity. The true beauty of this book lies in its versatility. You can open it at any time, on any page, and trust that you'll receive exactly what you need at that moment. It's an empowering tool for those seeking to evolve, emerge, and expand into their highest potential.'
~MICHELLE IRENE STUPSKI

'Jen is as intuitive, insightful and graceful in her written word as she is in real life. This guide is filled with profound wisdom, practical action steps and tools that anyone can use to transform their life. I love that I can use this book in a way that serves me in life as life unfolds. I now have a resource I can use to help shift my mindset. Thank you Jen, for sharing your gifts with the world!'
~SUE SCHUMACHER

'*Evolve, Emerge, Expand: Return to Your Authentic Self* has been my resource through the many changes in my life. Jennifer Kupcho is so relatable. Sharing her personal experiences, which serve to guide her readers back to their divine power. Whether you start at the beginning, middle or end, every choice you make will guide you back to your heart with a deeper love and multitude of grace for you!'
~GINA IANNOTTI

'Jennifer's book lets you choose your own path. It's a captivating read that gives you the tools to grow and remember your Authentic Self. There are prompts to journal and reflect & affirmations to help you dive deeper into your healing journey. It's a beautifully written book that will inspire you to dive inward and become your truest Authentic Self.'
~REBECCA DRUMMOND

'I love books, I am a huge reader. THIS book is amazing in so many ways. The content is thought provoking and helpful and full of real life examples. Jennifer wrote it and formatted it in such a way that I can pick up the book and go to a section of interest in that moment without reading all the preceding chapters first. Well done, is what comes to mind! Well done!'
~ANGEL ANN

'Jennifer has crafted a life changing, self-guided journey that becomes a soothing balm for your soul. This is a book for any season in life. I will return to this for healing and exponential growth again and again. Her unique approach to your inner journey puts the wheel in your hands as you navigate through your memories, your wounds, and more importantly, your healing. With every step—acknowledge with gratitude, release, and make room for the beautiful future awaiting you, unencumbered by the baggage, disappointment, and pain of your past.'
~JO-ANN WILBER

'Jennifer's work will ignite your soul and inspire you to go beyond your perceived limitations. Be prepared to be challenged and awakened. What awaits you on this journey is pure magic.'
~JODIE E.

CHOOSE YOUR JOURNEY EXPERIENCE

EVOLVE
EMERGE
EXPAND

Return to Your Authentic Self

Guidance for Reclaiming
Your Feminine Divine Power

JENNIFER KUPCHO

©2024

Published in the United States by: Emergence Publications
Cover and Interior Design: Jennifer Kupcho

All rights reserved. This publication is the original work of Jennifer Kupcho and was not generated using artificial intelligence. Every story and piece of information is authentically crafted by the author. Other quotes and footnotes are included with proper credit given. No part of this publication may be reproduced, distributed, or transmitted in any form or by any means, including photocopying, recording, or other electronic or mechanical methods, without the prior written permission of the publisher, except in the case of brief quotations embodied in critical reviews and certain other noncommercial uses permitted by copyright law. For permission requests, write to the publisher at hello@jenkupcho.com, addressed "Attention: Permissions Coordinator."

The author of this book does not provide medical advice or prescribe any techniques as a form of treatment for physical, emotional, or medical issues without consulting a physician. The purpose of this book is to offer general information to support your journey toward emotional, physical, and spiritual well-being. If you choose to apply any of the information contained in this book, please consult with a healthcare professional. The author and publisher cannot be held responsible for any adverse effects or consequences resulting from the use of the suggestions in this book.

Tradepaper ISBN: 979-8-218-49112-3

1st edition, 2024

To my Mother and Father

To my Mother,
The woman who has always led by her
soul and loving spirit. Who
showed me that anything was possible.
No words were ever needed; your heart-led
actions and unwavering belief in angels conveyed
everything with love and grace. Thank you
for showing me the power
of possibility in the feminine divine.

AND

To my Father,
The man who is grounded in his
healed masculine divine.
Who supported his wife and daughters in
every endeavor, teaching us that
no dream was ever too big. Thank you
for always calling me *Love*,
reminding me that *I am* love. Born from
love, to share love with the world.

CONTENTS

Your Personal Roadmap	ix
Pathfinder Quick Guide	xiii
Preface	xviii
The Compass for Your Journey	xxiv
EVOLVE. EMERGE. EXPAND.	xxviii

Evolve

1.1: Embracing Your Worth: Asking for What You Want	2
1.2: Choose Authenticity Over Approval	8
1.3: Transform Through Self-Discovery	12
1.4: The Magic of Embracing the Unconventional	18
1.5: Understanding the Non-Linear Path	24
1.6: Finding Light in the Shadows	31
1.7: Never Abandon Your True Self	39
1.8: Release the Need for Approval	46
1.9: Be the Architect of Your Happiness	51
1.10: Sacrifice Pain to Find Peace	55
1.11: Embody Your Unique Essence	62
1.12: Illuminate with Your Inner Light	68

Emerge

2.1: Be Your Own Permission Slip	74
2.2: Go Big: Trust Your Process	79
2.3: Return to Who You Were Created to Be	82
2.4: Be the Host of Your Life	86
2.5: Happiness is a State of Being	91

2.6: Embracing Imperfections	96
2.7: Life Happens For Us, Not to Us.	102
2.8: Embrace Your True Self: Lessons from the Arena	108
2.9: The Transformative Power of Momentum	114
2.10: The Power of Abundance and Gratitude	119
2.11: Regret as Your GPS: Course Correction	125
2.12: The Power of Healing: Emerge as Your Authentic Self	131

Expand

3.1: Choosing Courage over Comfort.	139
3.2: Claiming Your Happiness	144
3.3: The Power of Asking Questions	149
3.4: The Power of Belonging	154
3.5: Navigating the Journey of the Empath	161
3.6: The Ripple Effect	166
3.7: Subtle Miracles in Everyday Life	173
3.8: The Power of Imagination	179
3.9: Authentic Power and Peace	184
3.10: Crafting a New Narrative	189
3.11: The Power of Letting Go	193
3.12: Authentic Splendor: Boldness, Beauty and Abundance	198

Afterword	208
Acknowledgments	210
About the Author	213
Songs for Your Journey: A Musical Compass	215

...

YOUR PERSONAL ROADMAP
Introduction

Welcome to Your Journey

Welcome to a transformative journey designed to guide you back to a life filled with purpose and authenticity. In this book, you will embark on a path of self-discovery, healing, and personal growth. Each section is crafted to help you evolve, emerge, and expand, providing you with the tools and insights needed to reconnect with your true purpose.

The Reason You Are Here

We understand why you have chosen this book. You are seeking clarity, affirmation, and a deeper connection with your voice and purpose in life. You want to be seen and validated in your feelings and are tired of being told how to live your life. This book offers practical strategies to overcome these challenges and transform your life. It gives you the permission you have been looking for to trust yourself again. No one knows what you need better than you..

Through this journey, you will:

- **Release Limiting Beliefs:** Identify and let go of beliefs that no longer serve you
- **Heal Past Wounds:** Discover techniques to address and heal emotional pain and trauma.

- **Reconnect with Your Purpose:** Embrace your strengths and step into your power with confidence.
- **Cultivate Authenticity:** Develop the courage to live authentically and align with your true values.
- **Embrace Abundance and Joy:** Unlock your potential for creativity, joy, and meaningful connections.

How to Use This Book

This book is designed to allow you to choose your own path. Each part—Evolve, Emerge, and Expand—addresses specific themes and challenges. You can read the book linearly or jump to the parts that resonate most with your current needs. At the end of each segment, you'll find a reflective summary, an affirmation, a soul-to-soul message, key takeaways, and action steps to integrate the lessons into your life.

You have the freedom to break out of the mold of being taught to read front to back and feeling shamed for not completing a book. This is more than just a book with pages to 'finish.' It is a coaching tool to pull out whenever you need extra support. When you are called to a section that resonates with you, you will always be given more choices at the end. Simply choose the direction you want to go, look up the section in the contents, and follow your intuition to the next leg of your journey.

Want to read it from back to front? Go for it! Want to read it from section to section? You have control. Trust your intuition.

The **Pathfinder Quick Guide** at the front of the book will help you navigate your journey, allowing you to find the right chapter or section that addresses your current needs. Additionally, at the end of each section, you will find the **Path to Progress**, which provides ways to make immediate shifts in your life through affirmations, summaries, action steps, journal prompts, and more.

The Path to Your Authentic Self

The journey to your Authentic Self involves three key phases: Evolve, Emerge, and Expand. Each phase represents a stage in the process of self-discovery and personal growth.

1. **Evolve:** This phase focuses on letting go of old patterns and beliefs that no longer serve you. It encourages introspection, healing, and the release of pain to make room for inner peace and growth.
2. **Emerge:** In this phase, you begin to reconnect with your true self. You learn to embrace your strengths, confront your fears, and step into your power. This is a time of self-acceptance and the cultivation of courage and authenticity.
3. **Expand:** The final phase is about living fully and authentically. It encourages you to share your gifts with the world, create meaningful connections, and contribute to the collective healing and growth of humanity. This phase is about embracing abundance, creativity, and joy.

Throughout the book, you will find references to different sections that can guide you based on specific challenges or themes you are experiencing in your life. The **Pathfinder Quick Guide** at the front of the book will help you navigate your journey, allowing you to find the right part that addresses your current needs. At the end of each chapter, you will also find suggestions for two additional sections that you can read if the message in that section resonated with you.

By engaging with the content in this book, you will gain a deeper understanding of yourself, heal past wounds, and step into a life of authenticity, empowerment, and joy. Welcome to your journey of self-discovery and transformation.

PATHFINDER QUICK GUIDE

Welcome to the **Pathfinder Quick Guide**! This quick reference is designed to help you navigate *Evolve, Emerge, Expand: Returning to Your Authentic Self* in a way that suits your personal journey. Whether you want to read it from beginning to end, explore all the sections of *Evolve, Emerge,* or *Expand,* or focus on specific topics that resonate with you, this book gives you the freedom to choose. The era of being told what to do and how to do it is over. This is a self-help book for you, the reader, who wants to call the shots - including how you will read the book and gain the information you seek.

On the next page, you'll find a list of topics and their corresponding sections. Use this guide to explore the themes that speak to you the most and trust your instincts as you journey through these pages.

At the end of each chapter, you'll find a **Path to Progress** section that offers further directions and options on where you can continue your journey within the book. This approach mirrors the philosophy of living life authentically and trusting your inner guidance. Enjoy the freedom to read, explore, and grow in your own unique way.

ABUNDANCE
- **Understanding and Embracing Abundance:** Explore 1.9, Evolve 1.11, Expand 3.12
- **Shifting from Scarcity to Abundance Mindset:** Emerge 2.7, Expand 3.3, Evolve 1.8

AUTHENTICITY
- Living Authentically: Evolve 1.2, Expand 3.1, Emerge 2.11
- Striving to Be True: Evolve 1.2, Emerge 2.1, Expand 3.4

BALANCE
- **Inner Balance and Harmony:** Expand 3.9, Evolve 1.6, Emerge 2.6
- **Power and Peace:** Expand 3.9, Evolve 1.5, Emerge 2.9

BELIEFS
- **Challenging Limiting Beliefs:** Evolve 1.3, Expand 3.2, Emerge 2.3
- **Forming Empowering Beliefs:** Evolve 1.7, Expand 3.8, Emerge 2.5

BETRAYAL
- **Healing from Betrayal:** Evolve 1.6, Expand 3.4, Emerge 2.8
- **Self-Worth and Forgiveness:** Evolve 1.5, Emerge 2.2, Expand 3.6

CHANGE
- **Embracing Change:** Evolve 1.4, Expand 3.3, Emerge 2.4
- **Navigating Life Transitions:** Evolve 1.9, Expand 3.1, Emerge 2.10.

COMPASSION
- **Cultivating Self-Compassion:** Evolve 1.7, Emerge 2.2, Expand 3.6
- **Compassion for Others:** Expand 3.11, Emerge 2.8, Evolve 1.5

COURAGE
- **Choosing Courage over Comfort:** Emerge 2.1, Expand 3.5, Evolve 1.1
- **Bravery and Authenticity:** Emerge 2.1, Expand 3.4, Evolve 1.7

CREATIVITY
- **Nurturing Creativity:** Expand 3.8, Evolve 1.12, Emerge 2.9
- **Creative Living:** Expand 3.10, Emerge 2.3, Evolve 1.11

EMPATHY
- **Understanding Empathy:** Evolve 1.6, Expand 3.5, Emerge 2.5
- Empathy and Boundaries: Emerge 2.5, Expand 3.4, Evolve 1.8

FEAR
- **Facing and Overcoming Fear:** Emerge 2.1, Evolve 1.10, Expand 3.5
- **Fear of Rejection:** Emerge 2.4, Evolve 1.8, Expand 3.11

FORGIVENESS
- **Self-Forgiveness:** Evolve 1.7, Emerge 2.6, Expand 3.6
- **Forgiving Others:** Evolve 1.5, Expand 3.11, Emerge 2.

xv

HEALING
- **Personal Healing Journey:** Evolve 1.6, Expand 3.6, Emerge 2.5
- **Collective Healing:** Expand 3.6, Evolve 1.12, Emerge 2.11

IMAGINATION
- **Power of Imagination:** Expand 3.8, Evolve 1.12, Emerge 2.3
- **Creativity and Imagination:** Emerge 2.9, Expand 3.10, Evolve 1.11

INCLUSION
- **From Exclusion to Inclusion:** Evolve 1.3, Expand 3.4, Emerge 2.7
- **Building Inclusive Spaces:** Expand 3.6, Emerge 2.10, Evolve 1.12

LIMITING BELIEFS
- **Recognizing and Releasing Limiting Beliefs:** Evolve 1.3, Expand 3.2, Emerge 2.5
- **Transforming Limiting Beliefs:** Emerge 2.3, Expand 3.7, Evolve 1.8

MIRACLES
- **Shifts in Perception:** Expand 3.7, Emerge 2.7, Evolve 1.5
- **Seeing Everyday Miracles:** Expand 3.7, Evolve 1.6, Emerge 2.12

NARCISSISM
- **Narcissism in Empaths:** Expand 3.5, Emerge 2.5, Evolve 1.7
- **Understanding Narcissistic Traits:** Emerge 2.5, Expand 3.4, Evolve 1.

PEACE
- **Achieving Inner Peace:** Evolve 1.1, Expand 3.9, Emerge 2.11
- **Sacrificing Pain for Peace:** Evolve 1.10, Emerge 2.6, Expand 3.9

SELF-ACCEPTANCE
- **Embracing Self-Worth:** Evolve 1.3, Emerge 2.2, Expand 3.8
- **Journey to Self-Acceptance:** Evolve 1.8, Expand 3.6, Emerge 2.9

SENSITIVITY
- **Managing Sensitivity:** Evolve 1.6, Expand 3.5, Emerge 2.5
- **Sensitive and Empowered:** Evolve 1.7, Emerge 2.3, Expand 3.8

SURRENDER
- **Power of Surrender:** Emerge 2.11, Expand 3.11, Evolve 1.5
- **Letting Go and Trusting:** Emerge 2.6, Expand 3.10, Evolve 1.4

TRUST
- **Building Self-Trust:** Emerge 2.1, Evolve 1.7, Expand 3.11
- **Trusting the Process:** Expand 3.3, Emerge 2.6, Evolve 1.5

PREFACE

In this fast-paced world, where every second is accounted for and our days are filled with endless tasks and responsibilities, it's easy to lose sight of our true essence. We often find ourselves caught in the whirlwind of daily demands, expectations, and the unending chase for external validation. But amidst this chaos, there lies a powerful truth—a truth that can transform our lives in ways we've never imagined. By being intentional about what we truly want, we can reconnect with our core values and desires, finding clarity and purpose in every moment.

As women, especially those like me, in the second spring of our lives, we stand at a unique crossroads. Our experiences, both joyous and challenging, have shaped us into who we are today. Yet, it's also a time when we begin to question the paths we've taken and the roles we've played. It's a time when we feel an undeniable pull to reconnect with our inner selves, to shed the layers of societal conditioning, and to step into our authentic power.

Your Journey to Empowerment and Expansion

This book is not just another guide; it is a companion on your journey to rediscovering the magnificent light within you. It's a call to embrace your evolution, to stand tall in your truth, and to expand beyond the limitations that have held you back. Through the sections that follow, you will find insights, stories, and practical tools designed to support you in this transformative process

As you embark on this journey, remember that you are not alone. Each page is infused with the collective wisdom of women who have walked this path before you, women who have faced their shadows and emerged stronger, more radiant, and deeply connected to their Authentic Self. Their stories are a testament to the resilience of the human spirit and the boundless potential that resides within each of us.

The Power of Connection

At the heart of this journey is the power of connection—connection to yourself, to others, and to the divine. It's about recognizing that we are all part of a greater whole and that our individual healing contributes to the healing of the world. This is not a journey of isolation but one of deep, meaningful relationships that uplift and inspire.

You'll discover the importance of nurturing these connections, of creating a support network that encourages growth and authenticity. Whether it's through shared experiences, heartfelt conversations, or simply being present for one another, these connections will serve as the foundation for your evolution.

Embracing Your Divine Feminine Power

This book also invites you to embrace your divine feminine power—a power that is soft yet strong, intuitive yet grounded, nurturing yet fierce. It's a power that lies in our ability to love unconditionally, to create with intention, and to lead with compassion. As you tap into this power, you'll find yourself moving through life with a newfound grace, flow and confidence.

Remember, your journey is unique. There is no right or wrong way to evolve. Trust yourself, honor your pace, and know that every step you take, no matter how small, is a step towards a more authentic and empowered you.

A Personal Note

As a Spiritual Mindset Mentor and Emergence Coach for women, my mission is to guide women like you through this profound transformation. My own journey has been filled with its share of challenges and triumphs, each one bringing me closer to the understanding that our greatest strength lies in our vulnerability. It's in those moments of surrender, when we let go of what no longer serves us, we create space for true growth and expansion.

In writing this book, my hope is to share with you the tools and insights that have been instrumental in my own evolution and in the journeys of countless women I have had the honor of working with. May this book serve as a beacon of light, illuminating the path ahead and reminding you of the incredible power that resides within you.

The Journey of Writing this Book

Writing this book was a journey for me from start to finish, a process of breaking free from the norm and embracing my role as an outlier, a rebel. Traditionally, a rebel is seen as someone who defies authority or opposes the status quo. But I came to redefine what it means to be a rebel—not as someone who simply resists, but as someone who remains steadfastly true to oneself. To be a rebel is to continuously carve out new paths and think beyond the conventional.

For 27 years as an educator with a bachelor's in Special Education and a master's in Deaf Education, finishing my career as a Consulting Teacher for the Deaf in the West Milford School District, I was continuously asked to think of new and ingenious ways to approach situations. My passion was always to see my students not as their labels but as their true potential. This same passion and innovative thinking led me to write this book in a way that defies conventional structure.

When this book came to be, I knew it couldn't be done like any other book. It needed to have a sense of play, adventure and rebel nature. I thought of my students, how they challenged me to find new ways to connect with them and how their passion for learning inspired me. This book mirrors that approach—it gives you the freedom to read it in any way that serves you best. You get to choose where to start, letting your heart lead you and following your spirit.

The process of writing this book was guided by my Higher Self, my guides and my angels, leading me into a creative and exciting way of writing. Each section is connected, weaving truths from one to the next, allowing each to stand alone or blend beautifully with another. This mirrors our spiritual journey, which is never a straight line but a series of twists, turns, and returns.

In a similar spirit, I have a matching unalome tattoo with my daughter, symbolizing our life's path and journey to freedom. The unalome, a Buddhist and Hindu symbol, consists of three parts: a spiral, a swirl, and dots at the end. It is read from bottom to top, representing the journey to enlightenment. Our evolution is not linear but a series of plot twists, straight lines, and jumps. This book guides you to evolve, emerge, and expand organically, comfortably, and creatively, helping you return to your Authentic Self.

THE JOURNEY AHEAD

In the realm of endless possibilities, where rules bend and paths twist, a new story unfolds—a tale of rediscovery and a rebellion against the ordinary. Welcome to a world where words aren't just words, but keys to unlock your true essence.

Step into the adventure of *Evolve, Emerge, Expand: Return to Your Authentic Self,* where you're not only reading a book, you're shaping your destiny with every page you turn. Remember those books from childhood where you decided what happened next? Well, get ready to dive into a similar journey here.

Think of this book as your personal treasure map, guiding you through sections that each hold a piece of your truth. You can dive in wherever your curiosity leads, whether following a traditional path from front to back, exploring each section dedicated to evolve, emerge and expand, or selecting chapters that resonate with you. Each section stands alone, offering insights and revelations. At the end of every chapter lies a crossroad, where you're presented with two new directions to explore, guiding you on a journey of self-discovery tailored to your desires and dreams. Let your intuition be your compass as you navigate this expedition back to the core of your most Authentic Self.

Inspired by years of teaching and writing, each word in this book whispers the wisdom of experience and the joy of individuality. Forget about following the crowd—this is your chance to color outside the lines and discover what truly resonates with your soul.

After 27 years of teaching students who hungered for learning and growth but didn't all embrace traditional reading methods, this book is crafted to meet you where you are. We are simply our former selves, a touch taller, a bit wiser, yet often guided by the inner child within us.

Why not, then, extend a hand to that inner child in a style that resonates with her? This book is my tribute to that spirit of discovery and playfulness, inviting you to embark on a journey that nurtures both your intellect and your soul. From cover to cover, or section to section, the power lies in your hands. This isn't a regular book; it's an invitation to explore, reflect and embrace the journey back to your most Authentic Self.

...

THE COMPASS FOR YOUR JOURNEY
Choose Your Own Journey: Evolve, Emerge, Expand

Welcome to "Choose Your Own Journey," a book designed to guide you back to your Authentic Self. This book is structured uniquely to allow you to choose your own path. Each section—Evolve, Emerge, Expand—offers a different step in the journey, and you can navigate through them in any order that resonates with you. At the center of this journey is your power and choice, trusting yourself and your intuition.

Trusting Your Intuition

As you move through this book, remember that you hold the key to your own transformation. Trust your inner guidance, and let it lead you to the sections that call to you. This journey is about reconnecting with your deep, intuitive *knowing* that has always been within you, which society, limiting beliefs, fears, and traumas may have obscured. The process of reading this book mirrors the very healing journey you travel in life. It is not separate; it is one and the same. By choosing how to navigate this book, you are practicing the experience of how to live life, trusting yourself and your discernment.

THE THREE E'S: EVOLVE. EMERGE. EXPAND.
Evolve: Going Inward

Evolving is an inward journey, often misunderstood as an outward process. It's about returning to your heart center, stirring up the waters of your inner world, and seeing what rises to the surface. Here, you get to discern which beliefs, fears, and traumas are not your own and decide what to release. This section allows you to reclaim your freedom and sovereignty, choosing what serves you best. The Evolve section is about recognizing and questioning the origins of these thoughts and deciding whether to keep or evict them. It's always about you—your freedom and choice, not what others think you should or shouldn't do.

Emerge: Stepping Into Your Authentic Self

In the Emerge section, you recognize and release the limiting beliefs that have held you back. This is where you step into your true self, free from the weight of old patterns and thoughts. Emerge is about coming up for air, returning to your life with a renewed sense of self and authenticity. You recognize the limiting beliefs imposed on you, and are choosing to release them. This process is not about becoming something new but rather rediscovering your original, healed self. As you let go of what's been holding you down, you step back into your life as your most authentic self, realizing that this journey is about returning to your true nature.

Expand: Living Authentically

Expansion is the practice of living your truth daily. As you expand, you embody your most authentic self and hold space for others to do the same. This section is about walking your talk, radiating your light, and attracting others who resonate with your energy. The more you Expand, the more you create a ripple effect, inspiring those around you to seek their own authentic paths. Expansion involves practicing your truth in every thought and choice, holding space for others to shift with you. As you embody your true self, you invite others to see your joy, peace, and light, inspiring them to seek the same in their lives.

NAVIGATING YOUR JOURNEY

You do not need to read this book cover to cover. Feel free to jump around, exploring the chapters and sections that speak to you at any given moment. This journey is about you—your freedom, your choice, your evolution. Use this compass to guide you, trusting that you will find what you need exactly when you need it. The freedom to choose how to journey through this book is the experience and practice of how to live life. By discerning and choosing your path through these pages, you are mirroring the very choices that shape your life's journey.

Using the Explore Questions

At the end of each chapter, you will find *explore questions* designed to deepen your experience and understanding. These questions can be used in various ways, depending on what feels right for you:

- **Preparation:** Read the questions first to set the stage for the chapter.
- **Reflection:** Read the questions after finishing the chapter to reflect on what you've learned.
- **Meditation:** Use the questions as prompts for meditation, allowing them to guide your inner exploration.
- **Journaling:** Use the questions as journal prompts to capture your thoughts and insights.
- **Group Discussion/Retreat:** If you are reading this book with others in a book circle or using it at a retreat, use the questions to inspire meaningful discussions.

This flexibility in how you engage with the questions reflects the freedom and discernment that are central to this journey. In a time where you may feel that much is being taken away, this book and its questions are tools to help you reclaim your power and choice.

Let the adventure begin as you embark on the path to rediscovering the beautiful essence that is uniquely you. Welcome to *Evolve. Emerge. Expand: Return to Your Authentic Self.* Let your intuition lead the way.

Jennifer

...

EVOLVE. EMERGE. EXPAND.
You are returning to who you were created to be.

Until now, you may have felt that many doors were locked, denying you entrance and leaving you feeling shut out and alone.

You may have knocked time and time again, only to be met with silence. Without realizing it, you've set your worth based on silence and the absence of an invitation to enter. Your ego tries to shield you from the fear of hurt and rejection by others, but this fear originates within you. The perceived rejection from others ultimately stems from your own beliefs. It had you fooled – until now.

Now you are **evolving** back into understanding your truth.
Now you are **emerging** as the soul you came here to be.
Now you are **expanding** like the rings of a tree.

Each understanding brings about more expansion and growth. Each ring brings a new key of understanding, compassion and love for yourself and others. What you've been searching for all along has always been within you. As you continue to evolve, you will see there are no locks. There are no keys.

Evolving inward, Emerging upward and Expanding outward will bring you to your full truth. All doors are open and waiting for your entrance.

Each beat of your heart is connected to the integrity of the Universe. Your existence here is not random.

You knew.
You chose.
You are remembering.
You are evolving, emerging and expanding.

The now was the now before you knew the now to exist - yet still you trusted.
Yet still you knew.
And still your soul chose.

Your contract with the Universe was made in balance and trust.
There are no mistakes.
You are always the answer.

Lean in.
Answer the call for change.
Answer the call to remember.
Your existence is a beautiful pattern in the intricate fabric of the world.

Your soul chose this life.
You matter to the Universe, to every person and creature.
You are the answer to all questions.
Let today be the day you begin to live this absolute truth.

Evolve. Emerge. Expand.
Return to your Authentic Self.

SECTION I

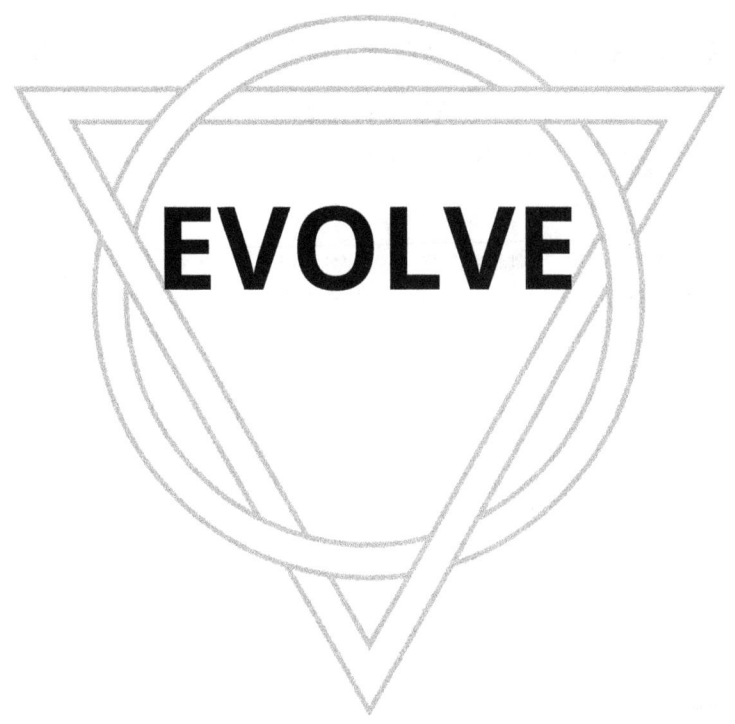

EVOLVE

1.1

EMBRACING YOUR WORTH: ASKING FOR WHAT YOU WANT

You are never too much, and you never ask for enough.

Contrary to what you may have heard, you are never too much. You could never ask too much from the Universe. You will always be enough for those truly aligned with you. If anyone has ever told you, "You are too much," I'm here to set the record straight: they were simply not enough for you.

When you align with your soul and flow with consciousness, the more you ask for, the more you receive. The more you receive, the more you can share with the world. The world needs you whole, healing, and sharing your gifts. The world needs your love, your voice, and you asking for what your soul needs.

Growing up, I never felt comfortable asking for what I wanted. Often, I didn't even know what I wanted. As I navigated these challenges, I learned to read facial expressions and body language well, just like you. In our very patriarchal society, it was implied with smiles and nods of approval (or disapproval) that good girls are seen but not heard. They were good if they were compliant and didn't ask for too much. They were good if they weren't greedy and were satisfied with what they got.

In 1977, I was seven years old and a fan of everything Star Wars and Princess Leia. That October, my mother surprised me with a handmade Princess Leia costume. Braided buns and all, I was excited to wear my costume for Halloween, but my excitement quickly waned when I thought about asking my neighbors for candy.

The force of the "good girl" was so strongly ingrained in me (apologies, I'm a bit of a Star Wars geek) that I didn't want to go trick-or-treating. The thought of opening my bag and asking strangers for candy made me cringe. I even thought about pretending to be sick, but lying definitely didn't align with being a good girl. Why did it feel so wrong to ask for what and wanted? Can you imagine—being afraid to ask for candy on Halloween?

It wasn't until I was an adult working with my life coach that I realized my fear of asking for candy was one of many signs that I didn't know how to ask for what I wanted in life. It was always easier to play the role of the good girl than to use my voice and ask for what I wanted. When others were happy with me for being good, it made me feel important and proud. I loved getting praise for my compliance. I loved receiving accolades for my offers to clear the table, wash the dishes, or help around the house.

To others, I seemed like a good girl, but if I am to be completely honest, my intentions were neither altruistic nor aligned with goodness. If anything, my choices were more aligned with being selfish. I needed their praise and hoarded their approval and love. Their praise filled the gaping pockets of fear within me and helped ease my feelings of unworthiness.

Let's be perfectly clear, *no one* ever told me I wasn't good enough. It was quite the opposite. I had a very loving and supportive family. When others told me I was good, it seemed to soothe my fears of unworthiness. I thrived when I heard them lovingly say, *Jennifer is such a big help* or *Jennifer is such a good girl*. These words filled my need to feel needed and loved. I developed a belief system that validated me when I gave to others and condemned me as *too much* if I dared to ask for what I wanted or needed. This insatiable need to be recognized as 'good' shaped my self-worth.

This belief also pushed my body into a state of dis-ease. It set my body on a painful path of migraines. It's no coincidence they started around age seven—the same age I began internalizing the belief that asking for what I wanted meant I wasn't worthy of love.

Every time I had a migraine, I was cared for and told to rest, which required me to receive love from others without needing to be a 'good girl' and earn it. It's crazy that I created such a belief, especially since love was freely given in my home.

Unconsciously, I convinced myself that I deserved love only when I was being helpful, which meant I felt unworthy whenever I rested. However, my body found a loophole through migraines, forcing me to rest despite myself. During those times, I received extra tender-loving care.

Can you see where I began to twist the message of love, giving, receiving, and worthiness? I subconsciously made a powerful connection between illness and receiving love. The limiting beliefs we create can lead to physical discomfort and actual disease in our bodies. I was only seven, so I didn't realize I had formed a belief system centered on not expressing my desires and thinking I had to serve others to be worthy of love.

TRUTH: We are NEVER too much, and we can NEVER ask for too much love.

Our body keeps score, and when we are out of alignment with our authentic truth (what our soul knows, not what our mind thinks), our bodies hold the pain. The dis-ease we feel surfaces in unexpected ways. For me, it was years of migraines and my body screaming what my soul knew to be true: *You're out of alignment. You're not too much. You can ask for what you want.*

My migraines were my body's way of throwing a temper tantrum to get my attention, but I didn't fully understand its message until I was ready to declare, *Enough is enough. I'm tired of feeling sick and tired.* This realization didn't come until I was nearly forty years old.

Through this journey, I began to understand the true meaning of alignment. Alignment, for me, is about embracing gratitude for what I already have while confidently aspiring for more. It's realizing that my worth isn't tied to how much I do for others but in recognizing and honoring my own needs and desires.

When I live in alignment, I give myself permission to seek and receive without guilt, understanding that my well-being and happiness are just as important as anyone else's.

More for us means more for everyone around us.
More faith.
More joy.
More laughter.
More peace.

When you tune into what your soul needs, you will be able to ask for more without feeling guilty. The more abundance you live in, the more abundance you will share with others.

Abundant thoughts.
Abundant love.

Abundant faith.
Abundant time.
Abundant happiness.

It starts with the release of guilt, fear, and shame around asking. Get clear. Release your fear. Ask and be open to receive.

PATH TO PROGRESS

Transforming Limiting Beliefs and Embracing Your Worth:

- ☐ **Affirmation:** *"I am worthy of love and care without conditions."*
- ☐ **Soul to Soul Message:** Understand that your worth is inherent and not dependent on your actions or the approval of others.
- ☐ **Key Takeaways:** Recognize how limiting beliefs can manifest as physical dis-ease. Emphasize the importance of aligning with your authentic self and releasing beliefs no longer serving you.
- ☐ **Action Step:** Reflect on a limiting belief you have held about your worth. Write down how this belief has affected your life and what steps you can take to release it. Then, write an affirmation that reinforces your inherent worth.

If you liked this message, you may want to choose your journey to Emerge 2.1 or Expand 3.1.

Evolve Exploration

What aren't you asking for that your soul needs?

Where can you be more clear with the Universe about what you want?

EMBRACE YOUR WORTH

You are never too much,
nor will you ever be,
a universe within,
aligned with your soul's decree.

Ask for what you need,
without guilt, without shame,
for the world needs your voice,
your love, your flame.

Break free from the chains,
of being just 'good',
embrace your worth,
as you always should.

Healing comes,
from within your heart,
ask, receive, and share,
a beautiful start.

1.2
CHOOSE AUTHENTICITY OVER APPROVAL
Strive to be true, not good.
"We become responsible adults when we become disobedient daughters. When we finally realize the best way to honor our parents is to trust fully the women they raised: Ourselves."
~Glennon Doyle

Medicine for the Soul

You will no longer be forced into compliance.

You will no longer be shamed into submission.

At one time you followed the path.

Their path.

It was the path of least resistance.

You slept through the process and absently conformed to the mold they poured you into.

You lived in the dark.

You yearned for the light within you to be ignited once again.

The light that could never be extinguished.

It was small, but not silenced.

You were patient.

You called in your strength.

You called in opportunities to stretch yourself, to remember and reconnect with your light once again.
You called in people and situations to challenge your beliefs.
You called in love and stinging medicine to ignite your fire.
To slash and burn your fields so your crops would flourish and grow more bountiful than before.
To provide you with Phoenix Rising moments.
Your dimming switch has been dissolved.
You add oxygen to burn brighter and bolder.
Your light is no longer a single dancing flame.
Your light seeks to join the light of others who encourage you to be true, not just good.
People who value their comfort over your truth have not earned your approval.
Those who recognize the strength and worth of your Authentic Self have earned a seat at your table..
Continue to unite your light with others.
Return to the beacon you were created to be.
Welcome home. You are now remembering your purpose.
To be the light you've always been.
To illuminate the path of ease and flow and love and joy; for you and for the world.
To float in abundance and jubilation.

You choose!
No longer will you allow yourself to be forced into compliance.

No longer will you allow yourself to be shamed into submission.

You are returning to your Authentic Self.

You are remembering your truth.

Stand in your power.

Choose to be true to yourself, not good for others.

PATH TO PROGRESS

Choose Authenticity Over Approval:

- ☐ **Affirmation:** *"I choose to be true to myself, not just good for others."*
- ☐ **Soul to Soul Message**: Strive to be true, not good. Trust fully the person you were born to be.
- ☐ **Key Takeaways**: Highlight the importance of choosing authenticity over seeking approval. Emphasize the power of self-trust and honoring your true self.
- ☐ **Action Step**: Reflect on areas in your life where you have sought approval over authenticity. Write down one change you will make to prioritize being true to yourself.

If you liked this message you may want to choose your journey to Emerge 2.2 or Expand 3.2.

Evolve Exploration

Where in your life have you chosen to be good, not true?

Recognize your growth and if needed, forgive yourself for your choices in the past.
You needed to be where you were in order to expand.

I HONOR MY AUTHENTIC SELF AND CHOOSE TRUTH OVER COMPLIANCE.

1.3

THE JOURNEY OF SELF DISCOVERY

Evolve. Emerge. Expand.

Growing up, I often felt like an outlier, as if I was standing with my nose pressed against the glass, looking in. What I didn't realize back then was that my loneliness had less to do with being left out and more to do with my fear of actually being included.

There were also times when I wasn't invited at all, a universal experience that triggers our inner child to create stories around our exclusion. For me, it sounded like this: *I'm not pretty enough. I'm not funny enough. I'm not thin enough. I don't have the right clothes. I'm not worthy of love.*

As a young girl, I would have vehemently disagreed with this current realization. Even now, my inner child occasionally stomps her little Mary Jane shoes and mutters, *This isn't fair. It's their fault I'm not being included. Why didn't they ask more than once? If they really cared, they would have invited me until I said yes.* This, of course, was the victim archetype in full force—a role I unwittingly mastered to the point of deserving an Oscar.

What I've come to understand now is the people who value their comfort over my truth do not deserve my energy. My light seeks to join the light of others who encourage me to be true, not just good. By understanding this, I began to align myself with those who support authenticity and mutual growth.

If only I knew then what I know now: **rejection is protection**. The situations and people I didn't spend time with were not of my highest good. The Universe always has our back, even when we think it doesn't. Rejection steers us away from what isn't meant for us and guides us toward what truly aligns with our well-being.

But understanding only comes with time. We must live forward to understand in reverse. I had to experience that pain to later dig deep and discover its purpose. Pain always has a purpose. It's never personal, though we often believe it is. Pain is a neutral response; it doesn't choose to attack one person over another. We make it personal by the stories we create around it.

By choosing to evolve inward and analyze our pain and the stories we've created, we can connect the dots to deeper truths, helping us emerge more whole and healed. This process allows us to recognize patterns in our relationships and break old cycles. As we heal, we expand our capacity to hold space for others to do the same. The more we heal individually, the greater our impact in healing the world.

As an adult, I've invested in coaches and mentors to help me evolve into who I came here to be, shedding light on the shadows of the stories and untruths I'd been telling myself. My shadow work revealed that I often declined invitations out of fear of feeling unworthy. In turn, the Universe mirrored my energy, perpetuating my cycle of exclusion. The law of attraction works by bringing us what we believe in and put into motion. I made choices, and the momentum picked up, with the Universe echoing those choices back to me.

Third grade, I chose: I was afraid to go to karate class. What if I didn't do it right and the kids laughed? My fear had me refusing to go to my first class. My parents canceled the program and didn't force me to go.

Sixth grade, I chose: I was afraid to go to the dance I was invited to. What if people made fun of my dancing or how I looked? I feigned being sick and my parents let me stay home.

College, I chose: I was afraid to practice Christmas songs in sign language with a performing group of interpreters. What if I messed up and they saw I wasn't good enough? I declined and blamed it on not feeling well.

In each of these situations, I initially said yes, but fear and anxiety soon took over, causing me to make excuses and pull back. The circumstances varied, but the underlying fear remained the same: I'm not good enough.

Engaging in shadow work enabled me to evolve to a deeper level and emerge more healed. I now recognize that my ego's attempts to shield me from hurt and rejection ironically caused more harm. Achieving clarity has allowed me to expand and become the mentor and coach I am today. I am able to create space without judgment for others who are encountering similar patterns.

As you heal old wounds and break free from repetitive patterns, you will continue to gain greater compassion for others grappling with similar fears, traumas, and pains.

> ***Evolving*** allows you to understand your truth.
> ***Emerging*** allows you to live as the soul you came here to be.
> ***Expanding*** allows you to cultivate greater compassion and love for yourself and others.

Applying This to Your Life:

1. Reflect on your pain points and identify moments when you felt excluded or unworthy. Notice the patterns and narratives you've built around these experiences. Challenge these stories and ask yourself if they are truly reflective of your reality.
2. Seek support from a coach or mentor to help you uncover and illuminate the shadows of your untruths. This external perspective can guide you in breaking free from self-imposed limitations.
3. Practice self-compassion by acknowledging your inner child and the fears that have shaped your behavior. Offer yourself the kindness and understanding you needed back then.
4. Take small steps to break old patterns. Say *YES!* to opportunities, even if they scare you. Trust that the Universe supports your growth and will guide you through the process.
5. Reflect regularly on your progress. Celebrate your growth and continue to evolve inwardly. As you heal, be present for others on their journey, sharing your experiences and offering support.

By following these steps, you can realign with your Authentic Self, break free from limiting beliefs, and create a life filled with joy, love, and abundance. Your journey to evolve, emerge, and expand will not only transform your life but also ripple out to positively impact those around you.

PATH TO PROGRESS

The Journey of Self Discovery - Evolve, Emerge, Expand:

- ☐ **Affirmation:** *"I am committed to evolving, emerging, and expanding into m yAuthentic Self."*
- ☐ **Soul to Soul Message**: Embrace the journey of self-discovery. Your pain has a purpose, and by understanding it, you can transform and heal.
- ☐ **Key Takeaways:** Highlight the importance of introspection and shadow work to understand and heal past wounds. Emphasize the power of evolving, emerging, and expanding to live authentically and compassionately.
- ☐ **Action Step:** Reflect on a specific pain point or moment of exclusion in your life. Identify the narratives you've created around it. Challenge these stories and write a new, empowering perspective. Seek support from a coach or mentor if needed.

If you liked this message, you may want to choose your journey to Emerge 2.3 or Expand 3.3.

Evolve Exploration

Where in your life is the victim archetype keeping you from evolving, emerging and expanding?

Where in your life are you giving the Universe mixed messages?

• • •

Breaking Through Illusions

Imagine standing at the edge of a vast field, feeling like an outlier. The glass wall between you and the world is but an illusion, created by fears and stories of unworthiness.

Break through that wall. Recognize that rejection is protection, steering you towards those who value your authenticity.

As you evolve inwardly, emerge stronger, and expand in love and compassion, your light will illuminate the path for others. Embrace your journey of self-discovery, for it is the key to unlocking a life of joy, love, and abundance.

1.4

EMBRACE THE UNCONVENTIONAL

The magic lies in living in the inverse of normal.

Webster's dictionary defines the word *normal* as conforming to a standard; usual, typical, or expected. If you were to ask a middle school student what their definition of the word normal is, they would probably add, *to fit in*.

When I was a classroom teacher, I observed some students trying to fit in by being 'normal', while others stood out and acted indifferent to societal norms. One might think the kids who attempted to be different would resist the idea of fitting in, but they too found their own circles of friends and blended in.

They found other kids who thought similarly, dressed similarly, and shared their beliefs. Why? Because they wanted to fit in. They sought acceptance just like the "normal" kids. What the kids didn't understand is that they were all searching for a place to belong, not just to fit in. Belonging means being embraced for who you are, not for what you need to change in order to fit in. This is what humans crave. We are a species that needs connection to fully thrive.

If you were to look beyond the surface, you would see that the students attempting to show up in the rebel archetype with purple hair and piercings were no different from Webster's definition of normal. In middle school, adolescents strive to fit in and be accepted; some with fitting-in behaviors and others with stand-out behaviors.

Normal is relative to the person using the word. It is directly connected to the experiences they've lived through and the possible painful judgments they may have internalized in their life. Life is not linear, and sometimes we get stuck at different stages. Although it looks like we are moving from point A to point B in a direct line, we may revisit a lesson from our childhood because we haven't learned all we need from it or we haven't made peace with it yet.

Our language has power, and in the English language, normal is a very loaded word. It shows up in the dictionary as a noun or an adjective, but for many of us, it can be so much more.

The idea of normal can show up as a roadblock, a trigger, or a deep-rooted fear of rejection. This is why I emphasize in the *Expand section 3.3* that it is crucial to get curious and ask yourself more questions. *What does normal mean to me? Why is it important for me to be seen as normal? What kinds of feelings does not being normal bring up in me?*

As you ask more questions, you open more avenues to embrace and evolve into your true self—your Authentic Self. The person you came here to be, without fear of rejection.

This clarity will help you see you've been living in a self-made prison created through your attempts to live up to your definition of normal. Your cell door was never locked; you could leave at any time. All you needed was a willingness to live in the inverse of normal to slide it open.

Living in the inverse of normal is where you rediscover your magic. The magic where there is no drive to fit in. Where there is no fear of rejection. There is only authenticity, truth, creativeness, adventure, exploration, and trust.

When you stop conforming to the opinions of others, you release restrictions you've placed on yourself. If the definition of normal includes usual, typical, and expected, then the inverse of normal would be unusual, creative, and unexpected.

Imagine what a 'normal' (mundane) day would be like if you were presented with an unexpected surprise? Maybe you get a phone call from your best friend, or someone buys you flowers, or a coworker brings in donuts. This is the inverse of normal. This is unexpected. This is where you will experience pockets of magic.

If change is challenging for you, try introducing the inverse of normal into your life in small doses. Consider taking a different route to work, sitting in a different seat at the dinner table, or wearing a color you wouldn't normally choose. Each action will encourage you to slide open the bars you've been living behind and support your evolution into the most authentic version of yourself.

Applying This to Your Life

1. Reflect on your own definition of normal and how it has influenced your actions and beliefs. Ask yourself: *What does normal mean to me? Why do I feel the need to conform to it? What feelings arise when I consider not being normal?*
2. Challenge your current narratives by trying something outside your usual routine. Take small steps to introduce the inverse of normal into your life. Wear a bold color, try a new hobby, or take a different route to work. Notice how these small changes make you feel.
3. Seek out environments and relationships where you feel a sense of belonging rather than just fitting in. Surround yourself with people who accept you for who you are, without the need for you to conform.

4. Reflect on your progress and celebrate your unique journey. As you continue to embrace the inverse of normal, you will find yourself evolving, emerging, and expanding into your most Authentic Self. This journey will not only transform your life but also inspire others to do the same.
5. Step into the magic of living in the inverse of normal. Rediscover your creativity, your adventure, and your true self.

PATH TO PROGRESS

Embrace the Unconventional:

- ☐ **Affirmation:** *"I embrace my Authentic Self and the magic of living beyond the norm."*
- ☐ **Soul to Soul Message:** The magic lies in living in the inverse of normal. Be bold, be creative, and be true to yourself.
- ☐ **Key Takeaways:** Emphasize the difference between fitting in and belonging. Highlight the power of embracing your Authentic Self and the liberation that comes from rejecting conventional norms.
- ☐ **Action Step:** Reflect on areas where you have conformed to fit in. Choose one aspect of your life where you can introduce an "inverse of normal" action—something unexpected or creative—and commit to it.

If you liked this message, you may want to choose your journey to Emerge 2.4 or Expand 3.4.

Evolve Exploration

Where have you let others' opinions of you keep you locked behind the bars of acting, speaking and showing up as 'normal'?

Make a list of the changes you can make to return to living in the inverse of normal.

• • •

THE WORLD NEEDS YOUR CREATIVITY.

1.5

UNDERSTANDING THE NON-LINEAR PATH
Time is not linear.
*"Life can only be understood backwards;
but must be lived forwards."*
~Soren Kierkegaard

Life is a journey of self-discovery and growth, shaped by our past experiences of navigating shadows and embracing light. Often, life takes us to uncomfortable places, urging us to face realities that may not align with our ideal vision. It is within these contrasting landscapes that true learning unfolds.

As we explore the depths of our existence, we encounter a series of interconnected moments, each offering subtle hints of wisdom and insight. These fragments, though scattered and sometimes unseen, lay the groundwork for our journey. Taking that initial step into the unknown can feel intimidating, wrapped in uncertainty and apprehension. Yet, it is precisely at this threshold where faith finds its foothold, guided by the gentle nudges of intuition and inner wisdom.

Trusting the path laid out before us is like surrendering to a higher plan, where each step carries the potential for transformation. With every stride forward, we unravel the threads of our lives, uncovering the mysteries behind past choices and unforeseen encounters. Our existence begins to weave a tale of resilience and growth, revealing the subtle nuances and hidden corners that once puzzled us.

It's not difficult to find yourself questioning the 'why'. *Why did this happen? What did I do to deserve this?* We ask questions of life expecting an immediate answer, but that's not how it works. Time is not linear. We don't live life in a straight line, and it could be years before an answer finds its way back to your question.

We live life in cycles and layers. We don't travel from point A to point B as many believe. Our logical mind and linear masculine energy would be quite satisfied if it worked this way, but as I'm sure you have experienced, it does not.

There were vertices in my life when events came together to cause the perfect storm of pain and loss. Times when I longed to receive an answer, solace, and comfort. It was at those points where the *why* of it all escaped me. I was confused and found myself desperately calling out for an answer that didn't surface.

Here's what I've learned and now know to be true: **life happens for us, not to us.** When we find ourselves in the shadowy hollows and grief-stricken moments, we want immediate answers and an understanding of why. What we forget is that we aren't equipped to handle it all at once. But the good news is we don't need to, just as we will never need to go it alone. We are always protected, guided, and supported to evolve, emerge, and expand through the timeline we choose for ourselves.

Just as a three-year-old hasn't grown enough to ride a two-wheeler because their feet can't reach the pedals, it is the same for our growth. We are ready only when we have learned and shifted enough to make room to receive more.

If I asked you to look back from where you stand now to gain an understanding of what you questioned in the past, could you do it? I am positive you could. Looking back, you would be able to see how the pieces of your life's puzzle have come together to create a clearer picture. The same pieces that once seemed jagged and confusing now have softer edges and are aligned to fit.

Evolving into a deeper version of yourself allows you to look back at the layers of your life and understand why you couldn't comprehend certain things at the time. For example, as you evolve, you might now find yourself ready to look back and understand why the relationship you once believed was perfect needed to end. Similarly, you might gain clarity on why you didn't get the job you thought would change your life. Remember, everything happens for us, not to us.

Through it all, we continue our momentum forward to receive the gift of clarity. Enlightenment comes when we have evolved to the point of living through trust and faith. We do not need to relive the pain or experience the trauma again in order to understand what it taught us. We need only the willingness to digest the lessons we received.

Here is another important truth to know: we live in layers of experiences throughout our life. They do not arrive one after another in a linear fashion. Have you ever noticed yourself repeating a pattern? It could be a trigger of unworthiness that sets you off, dating a certain type of person, or stepping into a new job that repeats an old pattern. That's because you are seeking additional information about yourself at a more advanced layer of what you previously learned.

You are very familiar with learning in layers. You did it throughout your school years. Just as you learned in advanced layers of the same subject—addition, then multiplication, algebra, and trigonometry—you will continue to learn and evolve through the layers of your life.

The best way I can explain how to shift from linear thinking to recognizing your layers is to see it through the eyes of a student. Think back to your elementary years. Do you remember when your teacher used transparencies on an overhead projector? (I am definitely dating myself now.) Your life consists of those same transparencies.

Now imagine pictures on those transparencies, one atop the other. You begin collecting them the day you were born. Throughout your life, you look up at the board to see all the layers blending together to form a complete picture. Maybe there is a detailed snow scene projected on the board: mountains in the back, snow on the ground, a little log cabin with a wreath on the door and smoke coming out of the chimney, a family, a dog, a small pond with skaters, a fire pit with people roasting marshmallows—you get the picture.

The picture on the board is a compilation of all the layers of your life's transparencies. You can see the sum of the parts of your layers. If you would like to examine your life in reverse, you can remove one picture at a time. One sheet may only have a picture of a dog. Another may have the mountains, or a mitten, or a door, or a chimney. Alone, the transparencies seem bare and maybe a bit confusing, but together they create the completed picture of your life.

By looking at your layers and appreciating what you've experienced, you evolve deeper into the person you came here to be. Enlightenment and evolution of your soul comes from patience, trust, and faith in your layers.

The beauty of where you are in your evolution is you get to teach the next generation how to recognize their life in layers. You are here to help them dismantle the belief that life is linear. With your support, they will move through their lessons faster than you did and surpass your growth and expansion.

REAL-TIME

Recently, my 21-year-old daughter, Ashlyn Faith, called to share how she recognized in real-time a new layer of her life. Her sorority was taking on new members, and she volunteered to interview candidates. She was happy with the list of girls she was given because she felt comfortable already having met them.

At the last minute, she was handed a new list of girls. At first, she was sad, but she quickly realigned because she too knows that life happens for her, not to her. Ashlyn Faith opened her heart with a willingness to receive the list the Universe hand-picked for her—the list that superseded the sorority's choice of interviewees.

The Universe saw her growth and her ability to tap into her Authentic Self, and in response, sent her a soul who aligned with her frequency of light. She was ready to receive someone who was a reflection of her healing, of who she was expanding into.

In the interview, the candidate openly shared her love of sound healing, Reiki, and feeling like an outlier in her life since most people didn't understand her passions. But Ashlyn did understand and fully connected. Years of helping me run my women's retreats opened her up to be the student of all things personal growth and healing. Because Ashlyn trusted her layers and evolution of healing, she stepped further into her authentic truth, which allowed the new soul to find her. By practicing the deep exploration of evolving, she is discovering what it's like to be the host of her life and call in her tribe.

Evolution is choosing to move through life with faith that the entire picture will be revealed when we are ready to receive it. Through trust, faith, and allowing yourself to receive, you are evolving into the you, you came here to be.

These are the gifts you give yourself as you move through life, trusting and knowing that life happens for you, not to you. You understand life is not linear and each layer of your life has purpose. Trust them as they build upon each other. The light of your true evolution and enlightenment will always shine through.

Applying This to Your Life

1. Reflect on your life and notice the patterns that have shaped your experiences. Understand that life is not linear, but rather a series of layers that build upon each other.
2. When you encounter a challenging situation, ask yourself what layer you might be revisiting. What new insights can you gain from this experience? Embrace the lessons each layer presents.
3. Trust the timing of your growth. Just as a three-year-old is not ready for a two-wheeler, you are ready for each new layer only when you have learned enough and shifted enough to receive more.
4. Look back at your life from where you stand now. Notice how the pieces of your life's puzzle have come together, creating a clearer picture. Understand that the same pieces that once seemed jagged and confusing now fit together perfectly.
5. Allow yourself to evolve deeper into your Authentic Self. Know that each layer of your life is necessary for your growth and enlightenment. Celebrate the journey and the person you are becoming.
6. By embracing the layers of your life, you will find that each experience, whether joyful or painful, contributes to your growth and evolution. Trust in the process and know that you are exactly where you need to be.

PATH TO PROGRESS

Understanding Life's Non-Linear Path:

- **Affirmation:** *"I trust the layers of my life, knowing each one brings me closer to my true self."*
- **Soul to Soul Message:** Life happens for us, not to us. Trust that every experience, whether joyful or painful, contributes to your growth and understanding.
- **Key Takeaways:** Emphasize the importance of viewing life as a series of interconnected moments rather than a straight path. Highlight the value of patience, trust, and recognizing the purpose behind each layer of experience.
- **Action Step:** Reflect on past experiences that were painful or confusing at the time. Identify the lessons and growth that emerged from those moments. Write down how these experiences have contributed to who you are today and the insights they have provided.

If you liked this message, you may want to choose your journey to Emerge 2.5 or Expand 3.5.

Evolve Exploration

Where in your life can you recognize pockets of
living forward and understanding in reverse?

Set a simple and powerful intention daily: *Show me. Show me. Show me this or something better in my life.*
You will gain trust in knowing you will always receive what you need.

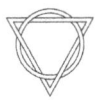

1.6

FINDING LIGHT IN THE SHADOWS

"The cave you fear to enter holds the treasure you seek."
~Joseph Campbell

In the journey of life, there are moments when we find ourselves walking through the shadows. These shadows represent the challenges and obstacles that test our resolve and shape our character. They are the moments of uncertainty, adversity, and discomfort that we encounter along our path. However, it is through these very shadows that we discover the true essence of personal growth and transformation.

As we learn to navigate through the darkness, we begin to illuminate our lives with the light of wisdom, resilience, and self-discovery. By evolving deeper into ourselves, we will see the transformative power of learning through the shadows and embracing the journey toward our inner light. There is a profound connection between our experiences in the shadows and the radiant light that calls us to remember our purpose and truth.

In our journey of evolving and understanding ourselves better, there is an undeniable truth that resonates with all of us. It's the awareness that within our own being lies both light and shadow. Joseph Campbell's powerful quote reminds us that the cave we fear to enter holds the treasure we seek. It's an invitation to bravely explore the depths of our own being, to examine the aspects of ourselves that might be uncomfortable or hidden.

Why is this so important? Because it is through facing our shadows, acknowledging our fears, and venturing into the depths of our caves that we discover the true gems of self-discovery and personal growth. It's in these moments of courageous introspection that we uncover the wisdom and strengths that have been waiting to emerge. As we embrace the practice of learning through our shadows, we not only experience personal growth and live through our light, but we also remember we have the power to shine our inner light on the world around us. In doing so, we illuminate the paths of others who are also on their journey of self-discovery and transformation.

In our relentless pursuit to shield ourselves from discomfort and pain, we often lose sight of our soul's purpose. Our ego seeks validation and harmony in our relationships, constantly looking outward for approval and forgetting to connect with our authentic selves. Life's challenges—whether in love, loss, or career—can feel like insurmountable obstacles happening to us, causing us to shut down and fear venturing deeper into the unknown.

But amidst the turmoil and struggles lies a profound purpose in our pain, especially as we evolve into our authentic selves. As we learned in *Expand Section 2.7*, instead of viewing life as a series of tests, we can shift our perspective to see it as an experience that *happens for us, not to us*. Embracing this mindset allows us to navigate the darkness and discover the light and vision that have always been present.

This shift in perspective became particularly significant during a tumultuous period in my teaching career. The profession's focus on observations and evaluations created a perfect storm for me to chase recognition and accolades. This journey provided many moments of deep reflection and growth. Continuous feedback and self-assessment helped me understand the profound interplay between light and shadow in my own life.

THE CAVE WE FEAR TO ENTER

During the twenty-fifth year of my career, through a series of challenging experiences, I found myself stumbling into the cave I feared to enter. Although difficult, this journey ultimately led to an epiphany: true worthiness stems from within, not from external validation.

As I began to advocate for my students, I found myself summoned to the superintendent's office, where I sat between my longtime friend and principal and a former student turned supervisor. Up until that moment in my teaching career, I had been the district's go-to person—always supporting after-school activities, earning exceptional evaluations from my supervisors, and even being nominated as Teacher of the Year. Given this background, I was completely unprepared for what awaited me in that room: betrayal, berating, and the stifling silence imposed by those in power.

Despite my dedication, I was reprimanded for being an innovator and thinking outside the norm for my students with special needs and high levels of anxiety. I had independently become certified and taught my students EFT (Emotional Freedom Technique), which, according to numbers and data, was increasing their state testing scores. But instead of recognizing the positive results, they feared my new methods.Instead of inquiring and embracing the opportunity to learn, they chose to shut me down out of fear of something new.

In that pivotal meeting, I was criticized for my actions and threatened with termination if I didn't silence myself and follow the rules. If I didn't choose to be a good girl, I would no longer hold a position in the school system I had worked in for 20 years. Somehow, I got through it without shedding a tear. I think the confusion kept me from breaking down—until I reached my car. That's when everything hit me at once. I spent the weekend crying and sleeping, grieving the loss of trust, friendship, and faith in my school system.

After a couple more days of crying all night and teaching all day, I decided to enter the darkness of the cave to seek my treasure. Truthfully, the cave felt more like falling into a rabbit hole, with me being Alice. Everything and everyone I trusted felt foreign to me. The betrayal felt physically painful. How could following my voice and intuition create such upheaval? I was sad but also a bit furious. I didn't understand why I was being burned at the stake for using my voice and standing up for my students.

With my heart pounding, I walked to the principal's office, feeling like I was stepping into a shadowy cave. When I arrived at his door, I could barely form the words in my head, and my mouth was completely dry. But I took a deep breath, swallowed hard, and finally spoke from my heart. Even though it felt like I was betraying myself, I asked how I could fix the situation and regain the admiration of my superintendent.

I met his gaze and poured out, *I feel like the superintendent will never see me as a good teacher again.* There was that word again—*good*. Before I could even continue and ask how to shift the situation, he answered, *He won't. There's nothing you can do to change how he sees you.*

In that moment, I stood with a foot in two worlds. One where I felt wronged, victimized, and devastated, and another where I felt complete freedom. I thought, *If I truly have no control over changing a person's view on my worth, then I am free to see my own worth without the need for validation of its truth. I am free to stop being a number and a value on an evaluation sheet.*

I was slowly remembering what I always knew to be true: what happened in the superintendent's office was for me, not to me. I began to see more clearly that what I witnessed in his office was about both of us. I saw his struggle to hold onto power over me, as he fought to control me and feel secure in his position.

I, on the other hand, was committed to keeping my power within me. I didn't need to win; my truth was too valuable to waste on him. That day in his office held my treasure—I made the declaration to stay true to myself and never compromise my integrity again.

When I ventured into the metaphorical cave of self-discovery, I initially encountered darkness and uncertainty. Yet, as I walked deeper into the shadows, I found a radiant light illuminating my path. It was in that defining moment—confronting my fears and staying true to myself—that I discovered true liberation and empowerment. Just like in ancient legends, the answers we seek often lie deep within the cave, waiting for the courage to uncover them.

The challenges I faced arose because I found the courage to advocate for my students and myself. I encountered resistance and criticism for speaking out, but I also discovered a newfound freedom in embracing my Authentic Self without seeking validation from others. The sting of their criticism brought me a deeper clarity.

I realized the pain and discomfort I had experienced in that situation had a greater purpose. It was leading me back to my Authentic Self and my soul's purpose. My soul did not need external validation to feel worthy. I had been so focused on seeking approval from others that I had lost sight of who I really was. But in that moment, in that cave of self-discovery, I found a light that illuminated my path forward.

I began to understand every challenge and setback was an opportunity for growth and transformation. And as I embraced this newfound perspective, I felt a sense of security and deep confidence in myself that I had never known before.

Just like Yoda said in Star Wars, *Sometimes we need to enter the cave to find the answers we seek*. Yes, I'm quoting Star Wars again—but it's true! On my journey, I discovered that the answers had been within me all along. I no longer feared the darkness because I knew the light within me was stronger than any external validation could ever be.

I emerged from that cave a different person, no longer afraid to be my Authentic Self. As I continue on my journey, I carry that light with me, illuminating the path for others still searching for their truth. By embracing my pain, I found my purpose, and by embracing my Authentic Self, I found freedom.

The journey through shadow and light is an ongoing adventure, a cycle of self-discovery and growth that leads us closer to our true essence. It is in the moments of darkness that we find the courage to explore, to confront our fears, and to embrace the unknown. And it is in those moments of illumination that we discover the strength, wisdom, and resilience that reside within us.

Life's challenges, no matter how daunting, are not roadblocks but rather stepping stones towards personal evolution.They are the catalysts that propel us forward, urging us to explore deeper into our caves of self-discovery and emerge as empowered beings, ready to shine our inner light on the world.

As we navigate through the shadows and embrace the light, we come to realize that the treasures we seek are not external but internal. They are the gems of self-awareness, self-acceptance, and self-love that guide us on our journey of transformation.

PATH TO PROGRESS

Finding Light in the Shadows:

- ☐ **Affirmation:** *"I embrace my shadows as opportunities for growth and transformation."*
- ☐ **Soul to Soul Message:** The cave you fear to enter holds the treasure you seek. By facing your fears and exploring your inner darkness, you discover the light of self-awareness and resilience.
- ☐ **Key Takeaways:** Emphasize the importance of acknowledging and confronting our fears and shadows. Highlight how these experiences lead to personal growth, self-discovery, and empowerment.
- ☐ **Action Step:** Reflect on a recent challenge or fear you've faced. Write down what you learned from this experience and how it has helped you grow. Identify one step you can take to confront another fear or shadow in your life, and commit to taking that step.

If you liked this message, you may want to choose your journey to Emerge 2.6 or Expand 3.6.

Evolve Exploration

What cave have you been afraid to enter?

How have you been focusing on being good, rather than true?

...

BLESSING OF LIGHT AND GROWTH

May you learn through the shadows, finding wisdom in the darkness.

May every challenge illuminate your path, guiding you to deeper truths.

May you live in the light, embracing your Authentic Self.

May your journey be filled with growth, joy, and boundless love.

May you always remember, that in the balance of shadow and light,

your true strength and beauty shine brightest.

1.7

NEVER ABANDON YOUR TRUE SELF

"I will not stay, not ever again - in a room or conversation or relationship or institution that requires me to abandon myself."
~Glennon Doyle

At the core of our journey through life, a powerful decision shapes our path forward. It's a promise we make to ourselves, echoing resolutely: *I won't stay anywhere that makes me lose sight of who I am.* As we navigate our experiences, facing doubts and pressures, a strong sense of self-worth rises within us. And as we continue to evolve into who we came here to be, we commit to honoring our true selves.

Each step you take reveals past choices and lessons. Exploring your innermost fears and joys brings clarity and growth. You now stand on the brink of transformation, embracing your Authentic Self.

As you dive deeper into self-discovery, you'll face the shadows of your past and the echoes of past decisions. To embrace your true self, you must confront your fears and uncertainties, facing the hard truths within. This journey is a deliberate step toward understanding what no longer aligns with your Authentic Self.

When you explore the depths of your being, you inevitably trigger shifts in your relationships. Some people may resist the changes in you, clinging to the familiar version of who you once were. Often, that familiarity was a facade, hiding your true self to meet others' expectations. The fear of disrupting the peace or disappointing others may have led you to betray and abandon yourself.

Courage becomes your guiding light as you navigate the path of self-discovery. Through the work in these pages, you are embarking on a journey toward your true, unmasked self. This requires facing the discomfort of introspection and acknowledging past mistakes without giving in to shame. By understanding that your past decisions came from pain and a fear of abandonment, you can start to forgive yourself.

In this journey of personal growth and awakening, we're all trying to find our way and learn as we go. Find solace in the recognition that self-abandonment is but a chapter in your story, not the final page. With each revelation, each moment of clarity, you inch closer towards the essence of your being, shedding the layers of falsehood to embrace the radiant truth of your Authentic Self.

Abandonment tiptoes in quietly. It's a subtle erosion rather than a dramatic explosion. It lurks in the moments where our silence outweighs our voice, where we sacrifice authenticity to uphold another's ease. Perhaps it's the laughter at a joke that rings hollow within us, a betrayal of our true selves as we drift further from our core. The internal fractures, the sense of disconnection within our own skin – these are the echoes of self-abandonment in service of others' comfort.

Have you masked your worth behind a smile that doesn't quite reach your eyes? Have you stifled your beliefs, believing them unworthy of voice? By reclaiming your narrative, you confront these buried commands, the whispers of self-doubt that nudged you towards self-abandonment. Exploring the depths of your mind reveals hidden, unconscious scripts that influence your behavior, exposing the beliefs that keep you tied to self-doubt.

This stage of awakening—evolving back to yourself—reveals the power of your beliefs. By recognizing and evicting limiting thoughts, you pave the way for transformation. Remember, change begins within; altering behavior without addressing the root cause is fleeting. Thus, evolving becomes a crucial step in self-exploration, where you rediscover your core, adopt new beliefs, and emerge more resilient and authentic.

Losing oneself isn't always about big gestures; it's in the small choices we make every day. Each decision, no matter how small, shapes our shared humanity, weaving threads of empathy, honesty, and connection that bind us together.

DANCING ALONE

For years, my daughter lived in the world of competitive dance, starting at the young age of six and dancing until she entered high school where she pursued a dance major. I became her devoted companion, aka "dance mom", driving countless miles to practices, competitions, and events in different states. Watching her glide across the dance floor filled me with a joy that lifted my spirit and made my heart soar. Yet, in the midst of the joy, there was a whisper of unease – a part of me that felt lost.

The world of competitive dance was filled with conversations focused on winning, where some families were consumed by the quest for trophies and success for their children. Surrounded by voices that valued achievement above all else, I found myself struggling to speak my truth, to stay true to myself in a sea of competition and comparison. The pressure to conform weighed heavily on my heart.

Surrounded by the chatter of judgments and expectations, I had a moment of clarity—a realization of how I had abandoned myself. In an act of self-discovery, I stepped back from the noise and found comfort in quiet reflection..

In those moments of rediscovery, I'd retreat to the sanctuary of my car, grading papers and listening to audiobooks. Sometimes, it meant taking a walk outside or getting a cup of coffee. And there were times at competitions when I chose to sit alone, aware of the curious glances and hushed whispers around me. They may have thought I believed myself to be above it all, but in truth, I was simply choosing never to abandon myself again. It was a decision rooted in truth, self-compassion, and a deep commitment to embracing my Authentic Self.

In competitive environments, I found the courage to stay true to myself despite external expectations. This journey required introspection, self-compassion, and rekindling my inner light. I learned that true authenticity means honoring your values, beliefs, and inner voice, especially when the world's priorities are different than yours.

Through this experience, I discovered that returning to your Authentic Self is not a one-time event but a continuous journey of self-discovery and rediscovery. It is a process of shedding layers of conformity and embracing the radiant truth of your Authentic Self. Each moment of choosing authenticity over compliance, self-love over self-betrayal, brings you closer to the core of your being.

We are the weavers of our stories and the architects of our destinies. It is in the moments of facing our shadows and embracing our light, that we find the true essence of who we came here to be. The journey of self-discovery is a sacred pilgrimage towards the heart of our authenticity, towards a life lived in alignment with our deepest truths.

May you continue to navigate the complexities of self-discovery with grace, courage, and unwavering authenticity.

May you honor the promise you made to yourself, to never lose sight of who you are, and to always choose the path that leads to your most Authentic Self.

In this journey, may you find solace in the whispers of your inner voice, in the echoes of your true essence, and in the boundless light that shines within you.

PATH TO PROGRESS

Never Abandon Your True Self:

- ☐ **Affirmation:** *"I honor my authentic self and choose paths that align with my truth."*
- ☐ **Soul to Soul Message:** Stay true to who you are, even when it's difficult. Your authenticity is your greatest strength and your guiding light.
- ☐ **Key Takeaways:** Emphasize the importance of maintaining authenticity in all areas of life. Highlight the courage it takes to stay true to oneself and the empowerment that comes from honoring one's true self.
- ☐ **Action Step:** Reflect on areas in your life where you may have compromised your authenticity. Write down one specific situation where you felt pressured to conform or abandon your true self. Plan a small, actionable step to reclaim your authenticity in that area, and commit to taking that step within the next week.

If you liked this message, you may want to choose your journey to Emerge 2.7 or Expand 3.7.

Evolve Exploration

In what moments have you silenced your true voice to fit in or avoid conflict?

What areas of your life have you prioritized seeking approval over honoring your Authentic Self?

• • •

YOUR PURPOSE IS NOT TO SURVIVE, BUT TO LIVE. READY YOURSELF TO RECEIVE AN INFINITE ABUNDANCE OF GIFTS.

AND SO IT IS.

1.8
RELEASE THE NEED FOR APPROVAL
What others think of you is none of your business.
"Exclusion is the most terrifying thing that can happen in our lives because it threatens our sense of belonging."
~Brene Brown

In high school, while my classmates puzzled over math problems, I found myself lost in daydreams of giving grand speeches. I imagined myself boldly standing in front of the class, not to talk about equations, but to advocate for more kindness and less drama in our teenage world.

I admit, it sounds a bit cheesy now, but back then, I was more of a silent observer amidst the high school chaos. Seeing peers judged for being themselves struck a chord with me. Even though I didn't fit the mold, I felt a tug to stand up for those crushed by stereotypes. I made countless speeches to myself in the mirror.

With hands flying and expressive facial expressions, I would silently mouth my passionate speeches to imaginary classmates in my bathroom mirror. These 'mirror talk' sessions were where I let it all out, championing causes in front of my own reflection.

Fast forward to adulthood, where I realize how those seemingly trivial high school moments actually shaped who I am today. While some of my peers chased the spotlight, I was always quietly questioning the norm.

It took years of courage and quirky self-talk to push past my fear of judgment. When I was in school, conversations about authenticity were definitely not the norm. You could easily find people to chat with about Madonna, Wham, or Boy George, but talking about being your Authentic Self—using a phrase circa the 1980s—would have been social suicide. Although I silenced myself back then, there was always a feisty spirit inside me, the girl in the mirror unafraid to speak her mind.

I understand the teenage version of myself better now because of what Brené Brown calls the ultimate terror: the burning fear of disconnect. *Exclusion is the most terrifying thing that can happen in our lives because it threatens our sense of belonging.* Sometimes I swear Brené sat in my Biology class or hid in my bathroom while I had my mirror chats. The dread of being left out, pushed aside, excluded from the pack—those feelings weighed heavily on me in high school.

Looking back, Piaget's dualistic thinking felt like living in a world of absolutes—black or white, yes or no. It was the *either you're with us or against us* mentality that cast a shadow over my teenage years. I desperately craved a middle ground, a space where judgment took a backseat and understanding reigned supreme.

Many kids get stuck in the first gear of dualistic thinking. But I was more drawn to the second gear - the incorporation of understanding, bringing together the shades of gray and the nuances that make us human.

Back then, my fear of judgment held me back. What if others saw me as different? What if I didn't fit in? The fear of exclusion loomed large, casting a shadow on my choices and beliefs. In retrospect, that's probably the reason I found solace in teaching eighth grade as a Special Education Teacher. Most saw eighth grade as a battlefield, but to me, it was a platform to break barriers, shatter stereotypes, and rewrite my past through my students' futures. I could give my class the tools I never had. I taught them not to let others live rent-free in their heads. And told them their real estate was too valuable to allow squatters to set up residency. They laughed at the visual, but they understood.

THE CHEAP SEATS

As Brené Brown would say, the people in the cheap seats are not in the arena. Those spectators hurling judgments from afar—they don't hold a backstage pass to your journey. It's not about pleasing the people in the cheap seats; it's about staying true to your path, unapologetically.

Looking back, I realized how often I had abandoned myself in my younger years. My true self only emerged during solitary mirror confessions and vivid daydreams where my voice echoed into the void. Over time, I came to understand that time was my ally, patiently guiding me toward a deeper self-awareness before I could finally release the grip of external judgment.

As I evolved and felt the whispers of regret, I recognized that I was exactly where I needed to be, even if I had lost sight of myself along the way. Each step was a necessary detour toward self-acceptance. The echoes of *I should have known better* gradually faded, replaced by a gentle acknowledgment of the past as a stepping stone to the present.

The regrets of the past serve as guides, leading us to the wisdom we carry on our journey today. When we embrace this, we see that the maze of adolescent insecurities and societal expectations was a transformative pilgrimage. For me, those moments spent in heartfelt mirror conversations and vivid daydreams were sacred rituals—a prelude to unveiling my true essence. They guided me back to my Authentic Self.

Now, in this part of our journey, we pause to examine the beliefs we've carried for so long. Do they still fit, or have we outgrown them? Have we mistaken judgment and fear for our truths? It's time to clean house, to clear away beliefs that no longer serve us, making space for those that align with who we are now.

So, from mirror whispers to real-world ponderings, here I am—sharing my journey of discovering and celebrating my true colors so you can too. No more whispers. Now, I stand tall, ready to declare my truths for all to hear.

Applying This to Your Life

1. Take a moment to reflect on your past. Consider those moments of insecurity and fear of judgment. Ask yourself, how have these experiences shaped who you are today? Are there beliefs that you need to let go of in order to move forward?
2. Engage in 'mirror talk' sessions. Stand in front of your mirror and speak your truth. It might feel awkward at first, but it's a powerful way to reconnect with your Authentic Self.
3. Identify the 'squatters' in your mind – those negative thoughts and judgments that don't belong. Evict them and reclaim your mental real estate.
4. Embrace your journey. Know that every step, even the painful ones, have brought you to this moment. Trust in your path and keep moving forward, embracing the shadows and the light.
5. Remember, the journey of self-discovery is ongoing. It's about evolving, emerging, and expanding into the person you were always meant to be. Embrace it with courage and curiosity, knowing that the treasures you seek are already within you.

PATH TO PROGRESS

Release the Need for Approval

- [ ] **Affirmation:** *"I embrace my true self and release the need for external validation."*
- [ ] **Soul to Soul Message:** What others think of you is none of your business. Embrace your journey without seeking approval from others.
- [ ] **Key Takeaways:** Highlight the importance of self-acceptance and authenticity. Emphasize that seeking approval from others can hinder personal growth and that true belonging comes from embracing who you are.
- [ ] **Action Step:** Reflect on situations where you have sought approval or validation from others. Write down one instance where you held back your true self out of fear of judgment. Identify a step you can take to honor your Authentic Self without seeking external validation. Commit to taking that step within the next week.

If you liked this message, you may want to choose your journey to Emerge 2.8 or Expand 3.8.

Evolve Exploration

What belief about yourself, inherited from your upbringing or past experiences, is holding you back from fully embracing your true potential?

What recurring negative thoughts or self-criticism hold you back and how can you reframe them to empower yourself on your path to growth and evolution?

...

1.9
BE THE ARCHITECT OF YOUR HAPPINESS
You are the bridge to your own happiness.

You are the bridge to your happiness.

It's time to take a step. Keep crossing over.

Happiness is your birthright.

We don't earn happiness through misery.

We don't need to experience pain in order to attain happiness.

Pain exists.

Sadness exists.

We need to embrace all emotions, not just the happy ones.

It's time we recognize that the belief system we adopted surrounding happiness is misaligned.

Pain and suffering alone will not open the door to happiness.

We were not created to suffer.

We have chosen to experience and learn through all human emotions, but suffering does not need to be one of them.

We were created to experience a range of emotions in contrast, allowing us to fully appreciate love, joy, and peace.

To continue the cycle of love.

It takes no work to be happy.

We need only *be* in order to be happy.

It takes effort to be unhappy.

We must work to become unhappy.

To think unhappy thoughts.

To replay old, hurtful stories.

To wallow in worry, shame, guilt, and regret.

It takes effort and work to remain unhappy.

Do you wish to return to a life of ease?

The life you were created for?

To live in happiness?

You can.

Choose something you can **stop** doing, in order to be happy.

You don't need to add more to your plate.

You need to do less.

It truly is that simple.

Choose one thing to stop doing.

Your lack of effort will be the bridge to your happiness.

Your bridge will lead you to the next and the next and the next.

Take the first step and continue to cross over.

You are the bridge to your happiness.

It's time to take a step.

Keep crossing over.

PATH TO PROGRESS

Be the Architect of Your Happiness:

- ☐ **Affirmation:** *"I am the bridge to my own happiness. I choose to stop what does not serve my joy."*
- ☐ **Soul to Soul Message:** Happiness is your birthright. Embrace the simplicity of being, and let go of the need to earn happiness through suffering.
- ☐ **Key Takeaways:** Emphasize that true happiness comes from within and does not require external validation or penance. Highlight the importance of recognizing and releasing misaligned beliefs about happiness. Encourage embracing all emotions, understanding that suffering is not a prerequisite for joy.
- ☐ **Action Step:** Identify one habit, thought pattern, or activity that contributes to your unhappiness. Commit to stopping this behavior for one week. Observe and journal how this change impacts your overall sense of well-being and happiness.

If you liked this message, you may want to choose your journey to Emerge 2.9 or Expand 3.9.

Evolve Exploration

What belief about yourself, inherited from your upbringing or past experiences, holds you back from fully embracing your true potential?

What recurring negative thought or self-criticism is holding you back and how can you reframe it to empower yourself on your path to growth and evolution?

1.10

SACRIFICE PAIN TO FIND PEACE

To gain the peace you seek you must be willing to sacrifice the pain you suffer.

Throughout my journey of self-healing, I faced moments where I tried to let go of old hurts—pain, anger, grudges, and harsh judgments. But no matter how hard I tried, it felt like I was hitting a wall. It was as if I was clinging tightly to things that only caused more pain. Why couldn't I just release what was weighing me down?

Trained in NLP and mindset coaching, I knew there was a hidden reason—a limiting belief I was repeating in my subconscious mind. With the guidance of my life coach, I explored the pain I had been holding onto. I realized it had woven itself into my life, serving a greater purpose within me than I had understood. Like an old, worn blanket, it initially provided comfort but eventually took on a life of its own and began smothering me.

Despite feeling suffocated, I resisted releasing it, much like a toddler unwilling to part with her security blanket. Little Jen clung tightly to her blanket of pain, reluctant to let it go. Ultimately, my pain led me to go deeper in self-reflection, questioning the connection between my toxic suffering and why I allowed it to consume me.

As I continued to explore my inner world, there was a dawning of a new truth within me. By holding onto my pain, I was keeping myself stuck in a cycle of self-sabotage. The familiar feeling of suffering had become connected to my sense of identity.

Who would I be without the feeling of pain and suffering? It was a part of my foundation. In a world where change is inevitable, my pain and suffering were solid and unchanging. I could rely on my pain. Even though it didn't feel good, I knew it would always be there for me. Our minds crave stories and structure. It doesn't matter how wrong the stories might be, we are comforted by having a roadmap to follow.

Wanting peace while still clutching onto pain led me to recognize the conflict within me. This realization pushed me to face hard truths about the stories I had woven into my pain. These familiar stories kept me playing small. Breaking free from these mental chains meant being willing to feel the discomfort of challenging the stories that kept me afraid to take chances.

This moment of truth was a game-changer in my search for inner peace—it meant being brave enough to let go of the past and embrace a new path of growth beyond old hurts. It had me exploring my personal understanding of the word *sacrifice*. For me, the idea of surrendering my pain felt like sacrificing something I had always relied on. Something dear to me.

The idea of sacrifice meant giving up something I loved, like skipping my favorite snacks while on a diet. We all know the struggle - maybe for you it's the salty chips, or the sweet slice of chocolate cake. It's hard! I was shocked when I realized I was comparing giving up my pain to skipping my favorite dessert.

What did this say about my view on pain and suffering? Seriously?! I had a difficult time rationalizing it in my head. Had I been cherishing my pain like something I loved? Had I been loving my pain? It felt surreal, yet undeniably true.

What I came to understand was my concept of sacrifice had been deeply interwoven with my reluctance to let go of my pain and suffering. Over the years my struggles had become ingrained in me, casting a dark shadow over my sense of self. They had morphed into a piece of my identity, a familiar yet burdensome part of who I was.

The thought of releasing the pain seemed like a daunting task. I feared the cavity. If I gave up the pain, what would fill the void left behind? Would it be possible for me to separate myself from the suffering that had become such an integral part of my identity?

FILLING THE GAP

This question intrigued me, lingering in my thoughts until a revealing moment occurred. Last year, my daughter came home from college to get her wisdom teeth out. Witnessing her journey through the pain, healing, and adjustment post-surgery shed much light on the complex journey of adapting and accepting.

As she struggled with the pain and absence of her wisdom teeth, her body and mind also had to navigate the shift. It had to find new ways to move and adjust and ultimately learn to live without what had once been a part of her. This experience served as a powerful reminder of the natural resilience and adaptability within us, urging me to reconsider my own attachments to past pain and the possibilities that awaited me on the other side of release.

In the months following her surgery, Ashlyn Faith's teeth shifted and the holes grew smaller. She learned to eat and live without them. She didn't wake up every day mourning the loss of her wisdom teeth; the pain subsided and she learned to live differently than she had before. This is the truth for all of us—the universal law of rhythm will always provide us with the opportunities to shift. Change is constant. We know this from birth.

WE ARE HARDWIRED FOR CRISIS

As infants, we instinctively took nourishment from a bottle or our mother's breast. However, even at this early stage, we faced the first of many crises: the transition away from this primal source of comfort. Each crisis in life presents an opportunity to shift and grow, never to return to our previous state of being. This ability to adapt and manage crises is ingrained in our DNA.

As an infant, cutting teeth is a crisis—pain accompanies the body breaking open to offer a new gift: teeth. Our body is designed to embrace this teething crisis. With a period of discomfort, our teeth continue to break through, allowing us to eventually introduce solid foods.

Our ability to adapt to this new phase with determination opens a new world for us. Baby steps (pun intended) are essential. In the beginning, our coping mechanisms might feel like soft, simple nourishment—like baby food. But as we face more challenges, we build resilience, allowing us to handle and digest the solid, complex challenges life presents. From infancy, we learn that life is meant to continually change and grow. Change is the one constant in life.

Just as Ashlyn Faith's wisdom teeth no longer served her, I realized that my pain and suffering were not serving me. I surrendered to my crisis and let go of what no longer served me. I trusted that my body knew what to do, bridging the gap to healing. And it will for you too.

Be the bridge to your happiness by being willing to release, to receive. When you are willing to sacrifice the pain you suffer, you will gain the freedom, peace, and joy you seek.

PATH TO PROGRESS

Sacrifice Pain to Find Peace:

- ☐ **Affirmation:** *"I am willing to release my pain to gain the peace I seek."*
- ☐ **Soul to Soul Message:** To gain the peace you seek, you must be willing to sacrifice the pain you suffer. Letting go of old hurts and limiting beliefs paves the way for growth.
- ☐ **KeyTakeaways:** Emphasize the importance of understanding that holding onto pain and suffering can keep us stuck in a cycle of self-sabotage. Encourage embracing change and the natural resilience within us to adapt and find new ways of living without the burden of past hurts.
- ☐ **Action Step:** Reflect on a specific pain or hurt you've been holding onto. Write down what purpose this pain serves in your life and how it has shaped your identity. Commit to a small daily practice that symbolizes letting go, such as journaling about your pain and then tearing up the pages, or meditating on releasing the hurt.

If you liked this message, you may want to choose your journey to Emerge 2.10 or Expand 3.10

Evolve Exploration
Where have you been holding onto past resentment and pain?

On a scale from one to ten, how much do you desire peace and happiness? It's time to let that outweigh your need to hold on to pain.

Divinely Magnificent

The only smallness that exists,

is your belief that you are small.

Release your fear to receive the truth:

you are divinely magnificent.

Sacrifice the pain,

that binds your heart,

find peace within,

let healing start.

Step into the light,

where shadows fade,

embrace your worth,

no more afraid.

The Universe sings,

of your radiant glow,

a beacon of love,

for all to know.

In your magnificence,

let your spirit soar,

divinely crafted,

forevermore.

1.11

EMBODY YOUR UNIQUE ESSENCE

Bring your flow wherever you go.

In the heart of the superintendent's office *(Evolve 1.6)*, I found myself at a crucial turning point, uncertain of which path to take. Unexpected realizations threw me off balance, and during this time of major change and upheaval, I felt a strong pull to be genuinely vulnerable and authentic. A sense of beautiful betrayal hung in the air, igniting a flicker of courage within me—a determination to reclaim my true self and embrace life's flow wherever it may lead.

When unforeseen challenges weighed me down, a moment of clarity broke through the confusion, offering a glimmer of hope in the darkness. In that moment where my past and future met, I found myself dealing with both uncertainty and the promise of change. It was a moment that demanded courage and vulnerability, a moment that challenged me to peel back the layers of fear and self-doubt to reveal the core of my true essence.

In the chaos of changing circumstances and unexpected surprises, a new path called to me—one guided not by fear or uncertainty, but by the steady light of authenticity. As I let go of pretenses and stopped pretending to be someone I wasn't, I found myself at a crossroads. I could either stay on the familiar but stifling path of complacency, or boldly step into the unknown, guided by the whisper of my own inner truth.

With each heartbeat, with each breath, the call of my Authentic Self grew stronger. It beckoned me to bring my flow wherever I go, to surrender to life's currents, and to embrace the transformative power of being true to myself.

In that pivotal moment of awareness, I realized that I had been neglecting to truly embody my own unique flow. I had unknowingly divided different parts of myself into separate personas: *the Jen who exuded confidence in coaching sessions and retreats, the Jen who shared wisdom through posts and blogs, and the Jen who stood before her students in the classroom.*

This division created a sense of disconnection within me. Although I often spoke about integrating teaching and coaching, I hadn't fully embraced the essence of who I was—my jean jackets with angel wings, boho-chic style, vibrant gypsy skirts, draping kimonos, long necklaces, and crystal bracelets. These choices were a reflection of my Authentic Self. This moment of awareness showed me that true authenticity extends beyond the separate identities I had tried to compartmentalize.

Every detail of my attire, my hair, and my makeup formed the intricate pattern that defined my flow and my essence. It was in the moment of being challenged, of being told that I fell short, that I realized I could choose to see a new beginning—a liberation, a return to my Authentic Self.

During the last two years of my teaching career, a transformation occurred as my circle tightened and my authenticity shone even brighter. Students began to see the real me, with some even admiring my unique style of clothing.

By embracing my essence and flow, I let go of the fear of standing out. This allowed my eighth-grade students, even those who didn't know me well, to embrace their own individuality and bring their flow wherever they went.

THE BOOK NOT WRITTEN

Through this healing journey of self-discovery and authenticity, a second realization dawned on me—one that led me to an act of courage and vulnerability: writing a book. My book. My story. Our shared experiences. The realization led me to write a book that you are **not** currently reading—a book that was never meant to come to fruition.

I wrote a book and five and a half chapters in, confronted the core of my words and the truth they held. I decided to delete it all. The book was titled *Bring Your Flow Wherever You Go*. The problem was, I wasn't in 'flow' when I wrote it.

Though I poured my heart and soul into the pages, crafting a narrative born from pain and healing, I soon began to sense a misalignment—a disconnect between the words on the page and my Authentic Self.

You would think my passion for the written word and love for language would have been enough to write the book. Unfortunately, it wasn't. I found I was not writing to the reader from my heart, but rather writing to the pages from my ego.

My need to be valued as a writer overshadowed my passion and purpose for writing. The words sounded beautiful on the page, but they lacked melody and authenticity through my heart. They had no audience besides my desire to feel validated. Talk about not connecting to my Authentic Self!

With this realization, I received a deep knowing that I was to delete all five and a half chapters of *Bring Your Flow Wherever You Go*. Deleting that manuscript, with its painstakingly crafted chapters and woven words, was a moment of reckoning—a moment of surrender and sacrifice. It was an act of releasing the past to make room for the present, a gesture of trust in the unfolding journey of self-discovery and my own state of evolving, emerging, and expanding.

The decision to let go of those words, to delete chapters that held a piece of my soul, was a transformative experience—a leap of faith into the unknown. Through the act of deletion, I embraced the power of surrender, trusting that from the ashes of what once was, a new narrative would emerge—a narrative steeped in truth, authenticity, and a raw sense of being.

So, as you journey through the pages of *this* book, know that each word, sentence, chapter is a testament to the courage to delete, to release, and to surrender. It is a gift of vulnerability, an offering of authenticity and a beacon of hope that urges you to bring your flow wherever you go—to embrace the transformative power of being true to yourself and to surrender to the currents of life with unwavering trust.

Applying This to Your Life

1. **Embrace Vulnerability**: Recognize that vulnerability is a strength. When faced with challenges, lean into your vulnerability instead of shying away from it. This allows you to connect deeply with yourself and others.
2. **Courage to Change:** Pay attention to feelings of misalignment in your life and muster the courage to take the path that aligns with your Authentic Self. Trust that this path, even if uncertain or daunting, will lead to greater fulfillment.

3. **Bring Your Flow:** Embrace the idea of bringing your flow wherever you go. Let go of pretenses and allow your true self to shine in all situations. This openness will inspire others and create a ripple effect of authenticity around you.

PATH TO PROGRESS

Embody Your Unique Essence:

- ☐ **Affirmation:** *"I bring my flow wherever I go, embracing my unique essence."*
- ☐ **Soul to Soul Message:** Embrace your true self and let your authenticity shine. Your journey is about integrating all aspects of who you are and bringing your unique flow to every part of your life.
- ☐ **Key Takeaways**: Emphasize the importance of being genuine and authentic in all aspects of life. Highlight how compartmentalizing different facets of yourself can lead to a sense of disconnection.
- ☐ **Action Step:** Reflect on areas in your life where you feel you are not fully embodying your Authentic Self. Choose one area where you will consciously bring your full, true essence. Take one step towards integrating your unique flow into that aspect of your life. Write down how this makes you feel and what changes you notice in your sense of authenticity and fulfillment..

If you liked this message, you may want to choose your journey to Emerge 2.11 or Expand 3.11.

Evolve Exploration

*Where are you looking for others to validate you,
but you are not actually showing them your Authentic Self?*

What does your flow look like? How does your style communicate your Authentic Self? What do you love about your flow?

. . .

1.12

ILLUMINATE WITH YOUR INNER LIGHT

Light attracts light.

As we come to the end of this Evolve journey, it's time to bring together all that we have explored and discovered. *Light Attracts Light* serves as a bridge, connecting the inward evolution we've embraced to the outward emergence of our true selves.

The importance of showing up in our flow—our full essence, our style, our spirit, our unique presence—helps us evolve inward. It allows us to acknowledge and confront the limiting beliefs that have kept us from fully expressing our authentic selves. It's about identifying what fears and doubts need to be evicted so we can shine our light.

The journey of evolution starts within. It's an intimate exploration of the heart, where we uncover and confront the beliefs that have shaped our reality. Many of us have been living with the fear of truly being seen, hiding parts of our essence because of the stories we've been told or the experiences we've endured. These limiting beliefs are like shadows, dimming the light that is inherently ours.

Think about the moments when you felt your light dim. Was it because someone told you that you weren't enough? Or perhaps you believed that your happiness was dependent on someone else's actions? These beliefs can be deeply ingrained. The first step in evolving is recognizing them. We must choose what needs to be released, not out of anger or blame, but out of a profound understanding that our light, our essence, is our responsibility.

This is how you reclaim your power. It's about realizing that no one else can truly dim your light. Yes, experiences and people can impact us, but they cannot take away the light that is inherently within us unless we allow it. Although this truth is controversial because it challenges the victimhood mindset that many of us have been taught to live under, this realization is both a liberating and empowering condition to practice.

We often blame others for dimming our light. But what if we changed that narrative? What if we were to take back control and acknowledge that while others' actions can influence us, the power to dim or brighten our light remains ours? This is a radical shift in mindset; one that brings immense power and responsibility.

As we evolve inward and strengthen our light, we also contribute to the collective healing of the world. Our light is not isolated—it's interconnected with the light of others. Every thought, every belief, every action has a ripple effect. When we heal ourselves, we send out waves of healing energy into the world. This is the essence of *Light Attracts Light*.

The law of attraction teaches us that what we focus on expands. By nurturing our light, we attract more light into our lives and into the lives of those around us. This collective healing is what will ultimately bring about the changes we seek in the world.

In this journey of evolution, we have explored the essence of our being, challenging the norms that have confined us and embracing the power of our inner light. We've learned to break free from the need to be *good* by societal standards and instead choose authenticity, exploring the beauty of living in the inverse of normal. We've committed to never abandoning ourselves, recognizing that self-love and self-acceptance are the foundations of our peace and happiness. We've become the bridge to our own joy, finding balance within and bringing our flow wherever we go.

As we reach the culmination of this section of our journey, remember that *light attracts light*. The light within you is your greatest gift, a beacon that guides you and illuminates the world around you. Nurture it, protect it, and let it shine brightly. By embracing our inner light, we not only transform ourselves but also contribute to the collective healing of the world. Your journey inward, evolving and reclaiming your true essence, is the most powerful act of love you can give to yourself and the world.

Many of us ask, *What is my purpose?* The answer always lies within our light. Our light is our legacy—the enduring impact we leave on the world, the essence of who we are that continues to shine long after we're gone. Let this evolution be the catalyst for living fully into your truth, radiating the light that attracts and nurtures more light. Together, we heal, grow, and transform, illuminating the path for others with our shared brilliance.

Applying This to Your Life

1. **Embrace Your Authentic Light:** Recognize that your unique light is your legacy. Reflect on what makes you shine—your passions, talents, and values. Embrace these aspects of yourself and let them guide your actions and decisions. Living authentically will not only bring you fulfillment but also inspire others to do the same.
2. **Radiate Positivity:** Your light has the power to attract and nurture more light. Cultivate a positive mindset and practice gratitude daily. Surround yourself with people who uplift and

support you. By radiating positivity, you create a ripple effect that enhances the lives of those around you.
3. **Cultivate Connection and Growth:** Together, we heal, grow, and transform. Seek out communities and relationships that encourage mutual growth and support. Share your journey and learn from others. This collective brilliance will illuminate the path for those who follow, creating a supportive environment where everyone can thrive.

By integrating these principles into your life, you can live fully in your truth, attract and nurture more light, and contribute to a world where everyone shines brightly.

PATH TO PROGRESS

Illuminate with Your Inner Light:

- ☐ **Affirmation:** *"I am a beacon of light, attracting and radiating positivity and healing."*
- ☐ **Soul to Soul Message:** Embrace your inner light and let it shine brightly. Your journey of self-discovery and evolution has strengthened your essence, allowing you to impact the world positively. By nurturing your light, you not only transform yourself but also contribute to the collective healing of the world.
- ☐ **Key Takeaways:** Highlight the importance of showing up authentically and embracing your unique essence. Emphasize the power of recognizing and releasing limiting beliefs that dim your light. Reinforce the idea that our inner light has a ripple effect, contributing to the collective healing and positivity in the world.

☐ **Action Step:** Reflect on moments when you felt your light dimmed. Identify the limiting beliefs and fears that contributed to these moments. Choose one belief or fear to release and replace it with a positive affirmation that aligns with your true essence. Practice this affirmation daily, and notice how it influences your thoughts, actions, and interactions with others.

If you liked this message, you may want to choose your journey to Emerge 2.12 or Expand 3.12.

Evolve Exploration

Recall a moment when your light felt dimmed. Identify the beliefs or fears that surfaced and consider ways to challenge them to reclaim your light.

Reflect on a time when you shone brightly despite adversity. Identify the inner strengths you relied on and think about how you can nurture these strengths further.

• • •

SECTION II

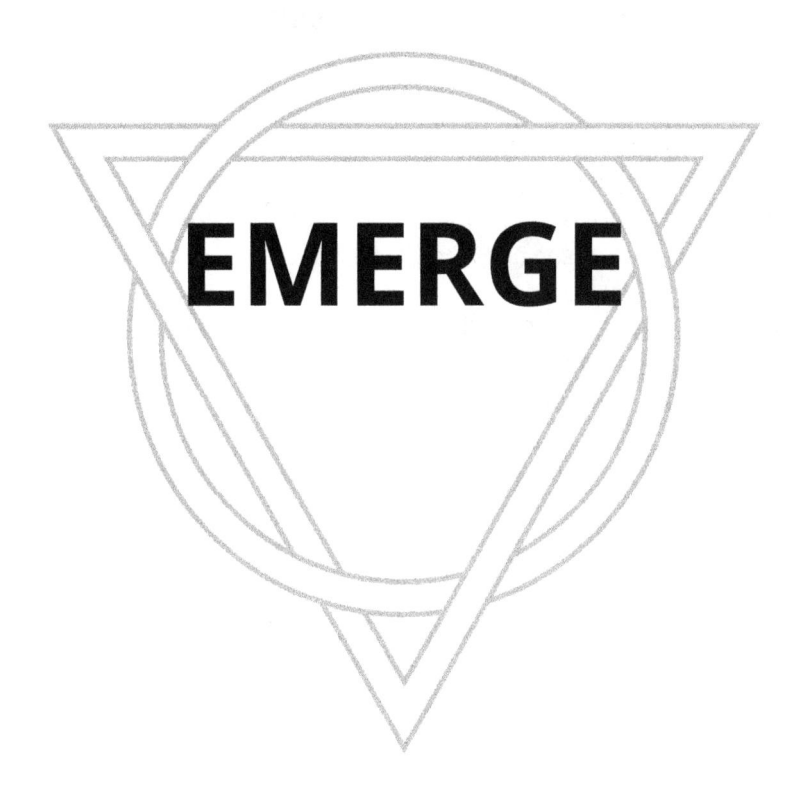

EMERGE

2.1
BE YOUR OWN PERMISSION SLIP

Knowing what you want and being willing to ask for it is the first step toward creating the life you've been dreaming of. However, to build the momentum necessary to truly take flight, you must break the conditioned beliefs and behaviors you've practiced since childhood.

Growing up, you were conditioned to ask for permission for what you wanted. Maybe your parents required you to ask for permission to ride your bike to a friend's house, or you needed to raise your hand for your teacher's permission to go to the bathroom. You learned early on that to get what you wanted, you needed to ask for permission.

While this served you well in grade school, it now holds you back from fully emerging into your life. I'll never forget the night my six-year-old daughter raised her hand at dinner to ask if she could go to the bathroom. It caught me off guard. Seeing her little hand in the air at the family table, asking for permission to do something so natural and necessary, struck me as strange.

She didn't need my permission. Reflecting on that moment, I realized how deeply ingrained it is in us from a young age to stop ourselves from taking action until we receive someone else's permission.

Asking and waiting for permission is deeply imprinted in us. We are taught that we are good when we ask for permission and bad if we don't. Shame is a huge motivator, guiding us into conformity and molding us into compliance. No one wants to be viewed as bad or to feel 'less than.' When we receive permission, it's like getting a gold star on our paper or a pat on the head for being good and following the rules.

Even as adults, most people still seek permission before taking action. When you pause and wait for permission from others, you break your momentum and interrupt your energetic flow. You impede your creativity, excitement, and inspiration toward birthing new creations into the world. Rarely do you ask permission from the one person truly qualified to give it: YOU!

You've been conditioned to believe you need permission to proceed and take action on your dreams. You may look to someone you admire, someone who has walked the path before you, to see what they think about your next step. But what can they truly know? They don't know your story from the inside. Only you know what is best for you. Only you can discern what will work for you.

When you pause to ask for permission, you're really seeking approval and validation from another. You're depending on someone outside yourself to decide your worth based on their belief system, not yours. You want them to tell you you're good enough to do the very thing your soul is lit up to do, and in doing so, you give up your sovereignty.

This indoctrination leaves you forgetting to trust your internal GPS. How can anyone who doesn't live inside your heart truly know what is best for your soul?

From a new relationship to a new car or a new career, you hold the power to manifest it through intention, passion, and aligned flow. But just as you can bring it to fruition, you can also hinder its arrival. Become aware of the power you hold to be your own permission slip.

You are the key. You alone hold the power. No more placing the power of your dreams and your life's purpose in another's hands.

Choose you.

Choose to trust your intuition.
The time for waiting is over.
The time to be your own permission slip is now.

PATH TO PROGRESS

Be Your Own Permission Slip:

- ☐ **Affirmation**: *"I give myself permission to pursue my dreams and take action."*
- ☐ **Soul to Soul Message**: Stop waiting for others to validate your choices; trust yourself, listen to your intuition and move forward with confidence.
- ☐ **KeyTakeaways**: Take a moment to highlight the importance of self-authorization and the drawbacks of seeking external validation. Emphasize that you are the best judge of your path and purpose.
- ☐ **Action Step:** Reflect on areas in your life where you have been waiting for permission. Write down one action you will take without seeking approval from others.

If you liked this message, you may want to choose your journey to Evolve 1.1 or Expand 3.1.

Emerge Exploration

What would you do if you had no fear of judgment from others?

What would you take action on if you knew you wouldn't fail?

. . .

BE YOUR OWN PERMISSION SLIP

YOU ARE YOUR OWN GATEKEEPER,

NO NEED TO ASK OR WAIT,

THE POWER TO STEP FORWARD IS YOURS TO ACTIVATE.

NO MORE LOOKING OUTWARD

FOR SOMEONE TO SAY "GO."

UNFOLD THE MAP INSIDE YOU,

ONLY YOU WILL KNOW.

YOUR HEART HOLDS THE COMPASS,

YOUR VOICE, THE SACRED KEY,

BE THE PERMISSION YOU SEEK,

UNBIND YOURSELF TO BE FREE.

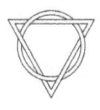

2.2
GO BIG: TRUST YOUR PROCESS

Big is listening to love, not fear.
Big is abundant.
Big is aligned.
Big is truth.
Big is authentic.

The world does not shift for you.
The world knows its size, its power, and its purpose.
The world also knows your size, your power, and your purpose.

Its ability to survive and thrive relies on your ability to trust the truth that you were created to go big!

Why is it so easy for you to trust the cycles of the world around you but not your own cycles?

You rely on the world's strength and truth.
You know the sun will rise each morning.
You have faith each evening the moon will wax and wane.
You know the tides will take their cue from the moon.
You know the fish will trust the tides.
You know the water cycle will allow the clouds to draw from the oceans and release when they are full.
You know they will share their sweet drops of nectar with the flowers and trees below.

All this because the world stays true to itself.
It trusts the process.
The world needs you to trust your process.
To trust that you were created with purpose, power, and magic inside you.
The world needs you to stand tall and not shrink your size to fit in someone's pocket.
Their pocket will never be big enough for all the tides, sun, moon, and healing water you hold within you.
Go big.
You were created for it.

PATH TO PROGRESS

Go Big:

- ☐ **Affirmation:** *"I trust my purpose, power, and magic. I embrace my true, expansive self."*
- ☐ **Soul to Soul Message:** The world needs you to trust your process and go big. You were created to shine.
- ☐ **Key Takeaways:** Emphasize the importance of trusting yourself and recognizing that each individual has a unique purpose and power. Highlight the parallels between natural cycles and personal growth.
- ☐ **Action Step:** Reflect on areas where you have been playing small or hiding your true self. Write down one bold action you will take to embrace your true, expansive nature.

If you liked this message you may want to choose your journey to Evolve 1.2 or Expand 3.2.

Emerge Exploration

Where have you been shrinking yourself to fit other people's limited views of you?

Go deep within to discover what fear is holding you back from showing up as your true size; your true self.

...

2.3
RETURN TO WHO YOU WERE CREATED TO BE
Carving Out Your Authentic Identity

Why is it that so many of us grow up and choose a career we aren't happy with before we decide to return to what we've always been meant for? For some of us, it's because we needed more life experience to tap into our passion. For others, it's because we were taught as children to stop believing in magic when we were still in the most magical part of our lives.

You may have been told by adults who were also asked to leave their imagination and spirited selves behind, *Get your head out of the clouds and stop being so silly,* or *You need to get more serious and decide what you want to be in life.* High school counselors administered career aptitude tests and guided you to believe you needed to choose a career that was financially secure and had longevity for the future. A job that would check all the boxes.

But none of those boxes were ever labeled:
- ☐ Lights me up.
- ☐ Makes me want to get out of bed in the morning.
- ☐ Fills my heart with joy.

And never did anyone tell you the average American changes careers between three to seven times in their lifetime. Why so many times? Because people grow and shift and emerge into their best selves after experiencing loss, trauma, and life lessons. The one constant in life is change.

One significant challenge in this journey of change is dealing with emotions that hinder our progress. Shame is the biggest deterrent to living a happy life, and it can be quite sneaky to detect. Shame can be given with a look or a lack of words when we need them most. And when we are shamed by the people we admire the most in life, it has the deepest impact on us. Consider a conversation where someone you respect is shaming you:

What? You are going to leave a job that makes you money just because it doesn't make you happy? Who cares about happiness? Shame on you for being so selfish and only thinking about yourself. You want to be an entrepreneur? There's no safety in that. How will you support yourself or your family? Shame on you.

SHAME ON YOU.

Shame is like hands on wet clay. It can form a new version of you while burying all your passions and dreams deep within itself. You could spend years wearing a painted clay avatar that is not who you were divinely created to be. One day blends into the next, and through it all, you choose friends and relationships based on your clay suit.

But this is not the end of your story. In fact, it is actually the beginning. Clay wears down, and the winds of time weather against your avatar until you remember what is at your core. Until you reach inside and find what has been waiting for you all along. It could be sadness from a 'failed' marriage or the loss of a relationship that has you feeling 'broken.' But broken is what brings you back to you. It is what has you cracked open to remember your magic.

This is not a midlife crisis as many like to call it. It can happen at any time in your life, and it is not a crisis but rather a rising moment. Just like hardened clay, you can be cracked into pieces.

You are cracked open to release your fear over what you will see within your heart. With love replacing fear, you will find what has been safely secured within the womb of your heart: your dreams and your passions.

And so your journey to returning to who you were created to be begins.

PATH TO PROGRESS

- ☐ **Return to Who You Were Created to Be**
- ☐ **Affirmation:** *"I embrace my true self and the journey back to who I was created to be."*
- ☐ **Soul to Soul Message:** Stop settling for a life that doesn't ignite your passion. It's time to reclaim your dreams and return to your Authentic Self.
- ☐ **Key Takeaways:** Recognize the importance of listening to your inner voice and pursuing what truly lights you up. Understand that it's never too late to change direction and follow your true path.
- ☐ **Action Step:** Reflect on the dreams and passions you had as a child. Identify any areas of your current life where you have settled for less than what you truly desire. Make a plan to take one small step towards reclaiming your authentic self and pursuing your true passions.

If you liked this message you may want to choose your journey to Evolve 1.3 or Expand 3.3.

Emerge Exploration

Where have you mistaken shame for guidance?

If money and other people's opinions had no effect on you, what would you choose to do right now? Would you change jobs? Travel? Volunteer? Paint? Move? Sit in this truth and ask what is holding you back.

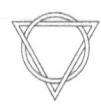

2.4

BE THE HOST OF YOUR LIFE

You are the host of your life.
Stop waiting to be invited to the table.

"Vulnerability is not winning or losing; it's having the courage to show up and be seen when we have no control over the outcome. Vulnerability is not weakness; it's our greatest measure of courage."
~Brene Brown

High school may be a distant memory for some, but if you are anything like me, you may have some deep wounds that don't feel so old—wounds that have taken up residency around being left out. I can remember cringing every time my gym teacher assigned students to pick teams. Why would anyone knowingly create such a hierarchy of power?

To the teacher, it seemed like an innocent enough request, but in my school, the result was always the same: two teams packed with the most popular kids, and a third that could pass for the *Bad News Bears*.

Two team captains always looked like they just walked off the cover of Teen Magazine. In high school, aesthetic appeal trumped athletic ability, and having a good personality held no weight on any of the teams. As we were being surveyed and found wanting, I was never comfortable making eye contact with the Teen Magazine kids. Fingers pointing, furrowed brows, and scrunched faces clearly expressed their disapproval of us—the outliers, the last ones standing.

Nervously fidgeting, I stood awkwardly in the center of the newly shellacked gym, waiting to be chosen. Palms sweating and heart racing, I silently prayed not to be the last one standing. With only two of us left, I somehow felt better if I was chosen rather than forced to join a team by default.

I think I prayed more on that gymnasium floor than I did in church. Period two's silent prayer was always the same: *Please pick me. Please don't let me be the last one standing.* Who knew gym class could be such a religious experience?

Well, winner, winner, chicken dinner if you guessed that I found myself to be the last one standing more times than I'd like to admit. I was the one with the 'great personality' who often had to be assigned to a team.

Reflecting on those moments, I now realize they taught me an important lesson about choices. We always have two choices in life. We can choose from a place of love or from a place of fear. The key is to live in an active state of discerning the difference. Love is easy to recognize because it is woven through our spirit. Fear, on the other hand, is tied to the ego and likes to hide in the shadows.

Fear often camouflages itself, making it hard to detect. I've seen how jealousy arises from the fear of lack, while anger often stems from the fear of losing control or feeling powerless. These are just two common disguises it wears.

Our desire to be connected, combined with our fear of rejection, can lead us to make choices misaligned with our Higher Self[1]. We bypass the spirit and operate directly from the ego through fear.

---

[1] The Higher Self is the wisest, most authentic part of you, connected to universal wisdom. It guides you with love and intuition, beyond the ego's fears and daily concerns.

These experiences highlight a deeper truth about human nature. Humans were built for connection. We were never meant to go it alone. Connection fuels our soul, and we gain enlightenment to emerge into our authentic selves.

Unfortunately, when we have experiences like the Teen Model gym class, we begin to believe being left out is more about us than it is about them. We want so much to fit in that when we are excluded, our ego creates outrageous stories telling us we are unworthy, unlovable, and will never belong.

The truth is, we all fear being the outlier. Ironically, this shared fear shows us we are the same. We are connected. The ego, or as I call it, *Little Girl Big*, doesn't want you to know this truth because if you did, you wouldn't let yourself be controlled any longer. *Little Girl Big* is the voice of our ego, formed from the big emotions and deep wounds of our childhood. She is the part of us that felt excluded, made fun of, and taunted.

As grown women, we may think we are making choices, but often it is *Little Girl Big* choosing from a place of pain and fear. If you knew the authentic truth, you wouldn't keep yourself small and hidden. If you knew the truth, you would be able to remember you've always had the power to be the host of your life, and you never needed to wait to be chosen by another to feel loved.

The Teen Magazine kids did not choose their teams from a place of love. They chose from fear—the fear of being judged, just as I felt judged in the middle of the gymnasium floor. The ego, or *Little Girl Big*, does not discriminate. It speaks to all women, keeping us small and hidden. But now you are remembering the truth, which gives you the freedom of choice. The freedom to choose again. The power to break free and no longer stay tucked away in silence.

Recognizing the voice of the ego, Little Girl Big, allows us to reassess the fabric of our lives, woven from threads of past trauma, and gives us the opportunity to choose differently.To shift our perception and unravel the stitches to create a new pattern and picture.

Not being chosen will never be about your lack of worth. People will choose you based on the amount of self-worth their ego tells them they have. No one outside yourself can define your self-worth. You were never undesirable, unworthy, or unlovable. That was a misunderstanding you believed from all the lies your *Little Girl Big* fed you.

The truth is you are safe to emerge as your Authentic Self. It is time to stop waiting for someone to invite you. To pick you. It is time to choose you. It is time to be the host of your life, set up chairs, and invite people to come sit at your table.

PATH TO PROGRESS

Be the Host of Your Life:

- ☐ **Affirmation:** *"I embrace my role as the host of my life."*
- ☐ **Soul to Soul Message:** Stop waiting to be invited to the table; choose yourself.
- ☐ **Key Takeaways:** Highlight the importance of recognizing one's power and not waiting for external validation to take control of life.
- ☐ **Action Step:** Reflect on areas where you have been waiting for permission or validation from others. Decide how you can take proactive steps to be the host of your life in these areas.

If you liked this message, you may want to choose your journey to Evolve 1.4 or Expand 3.4.

Emerge Exploration

What memories or feelings of rejection has your Little Girl Big used to make you believe you are not worthy of receiving love?

What pain are you willing to surrender in order to reconnect with your authentic self?

...

2.5

HAPPINESS IS A STATE OF BEING

Release the hold on the outcome. Untether the reigns and fly.

Emotions are typically short-lived and can be triggered by external events or circumstances. You might feel happy when you receive good news or accomplish a goal. However, this type of happiness is fleeting and can quickly be replaced by other emotions such as sadness or anger. Most people think of happiness as an emotion, but it's actually a state of being.

Happiness as a state of being is a more lasting and stable state of mind. It is not dependent on external events or circumstances but rather on an internal sense of contentment and fulfillment. This type of happiness is a way of being in the world. It is characterized by a sense of inner peace, joy, and gratitude that is not easily shaken by external events.

As a state of being, happiness is often associated with spiritual practices such as reading this book, mindfulness, meditation, and gratitude. These activities can help you cultivate a deeper sense of awareness and connection to your inner self, which can lead to a more lasting sense of happiness and well-being.

In this sense, happiness is not just an emotion but a way of living rooted in deep inner peace and contentment, regardless of circumstances or outcomes. The realization that happiness is a state of being is the powerful shift you have been seeking to free you from being dependent on the outcome.

When you tie yourself in knots and make choices from a place of fear, you hold yourself hostage. You allow fear to take the wheel instead of love. But remember, you are the sole proprietor and creator of your happiness. Now that you understand happiness is a state of being, you're ready to embrace the truth: your happiness is never contingent on the actions of others, your circumstances, or the outcome.

This truth frees you and empowers you to surrender to the outcome, while still feeling happy. You need not wait for something to work out before you allow yourself to be happy.

How much of your life have you tied to the outcome before allowing yourself to feel happy? So many of us are waiting to be happy......

> *I will be happy when... my relationship gets better.*
> *I will be happy when... my children are happy and settled.*
> *I will be happy when... I make more money.*
> *I will be happy when... I feel better.*
> *I will be happy when... I find my soulmate.*
> *I will be happy when... I can leave my current job.*

A significant portion of my life was spent in the 'waiting room.' I waited for life to start and for things to 'work out' before allowing myself to feel happy. I now realize that I put parts of my life on hold while tying my happiness to future outcomes. Today, I share with you what I didn't know then: happiness is a choice. It is not found in procrastination or the pursuit of perfection, but in living fully in the present.

DEMENTIA: I CALL BULLSHIT ON HAPPINESS

Recently, I had the blessing of spending a week with my parents. During that time, I experienced deep bouts of fear and pain, as well as joy and love. My mother, the most organized person I've ever known—the secretary to the superintendent of schools, who created and journaled photo albums for us, documented her grandchildren's firsts, made CDs of all our family movies, — is currently advancing in the stages of dementia.

Understanding dementia is like living in a different dimension. Up can become down, and left can become right. Or left might still be left, but gravity no longer exists. No matter how many books you read or how much information you think you have, your loved one is still shrouded by dementia.

They are not a textbook; they have thoughts and feelings, fears and love, inner-child work, and past trauma that surface throughout it all. What brings clarity at breakfast may no longer work by lunchtime. It feels like navigating shifting floors in a funhouse.

I found myself morphing into my mother's niece, long-lost relative, and cousin rather than her daughter. I felt the fear of the unknown shift every cell in my body. How could I ever be happy again? I very much wanted to call bullshit on happiness being a choice. How could I choose to be happy during all the chaos that was tearing my heart apart?

I felt frustrated and angry, calling bullshit on the idea that happiness was a choice. I held tight to my skepticism and waited for more proof. I allowed myself to feel the pain and fear that surfaced. I chose not to spiritually bypass any of my emotions. I let myself cry as a release, tap to recenter, ground by the ocean to restore my alignment, as well as meditate and journal. What I did not do was use those very tools to mask my emotions.Instead, I used them to lean in and feel all the feels.

THE SIGN

All feelings are meant to be felt, not just the good ones. So, as I continued to be like Alice falling down the rabbit hole, I also held on to a patch of earth and the possibility—my deep knowing—that happiness was a choice and a state of being. During one of my grounding sessions by the water, I asked for guidance from my angels and loved ones who had passed on. Specifically, I asked for a message from my maternal grandmother.

I half asked/half demanded (with love) and my guides didn't disappoint. Because I was open to receiving their message, it appeared swiftly. When I entered the house, I saw my mom dancing and laughing to her favorite Dolly Parton song, *Nine to Five*, with my daughter as they created new memories and TikToks together.

So much love. So many blessings. So much to choose to be grateful for. So much to choose to be happy about. Laughter. Connection. Joy. Love. New memories.

The question I was faced with was: Would I choose to untether myself from the fear of dementia and be happy by recognizing all the beautiful moments in my life, or would I choose to live in fear of the future? As I reflected on this, something shifted inside me. My heart received the proof I had been looking for. The choice was clear. I would choose to live in a state of being—happiness. And the happiness would carry me through the pockets of sadness and grief I would also face along the way.

In that moment, I vowed to continue to choose happiness. Not to allow myself to be imprisoned by sadness and fear. Sometimes there would be fear, but not all the time.

And I continue to choose to remember I have the power to let the sadness pass through me like a wave, not imprison me like a wall. I have the power to choose to release my hold on the outcome. I have the power to choose to be happy. And so do you.

PATH TO PROGRESS

Embracing Happiness as a State of Being:

- ☐ **Affirmation:** *"I release the hold on the outcome and embrace happiness as a state of being."*
- ☐ **Soul to Soul Message:** True happiness is a lasting state of being, not just a fleeting emotion.
- ☐ **Key Takeaways:** Highlight the difference between happiness as an emotion and happiness as a state of being. Emphasize the importance of inner peace, joy, and gratitude regardless of external circumstances.
- ☐ **Action Step:** Reflect on areas where you have tied your happiness to external outcomes. Make a conscious choice to untether your happiness from these outcomes and embrace it as a state of being.

If you liked this message, you may want to choose your journey to Evolve 1.5 or Expand 3.5.

Emerge Exploration

Where are you attaching your happiness to an outcome in your life?

Where can you choose to live in a state of happiness today?

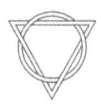

2.6

EMBRACING IMPERFECTIONS:
Live a perfectly imperfect life.

"Your value is in your imperfection. As you accept your flaws, you can transform them into tools for growth and self-discovery."
~ Wayne Dyer

In the sacred space of emergence, where shadows transform into light and mistakes pave the path to growth, we discover the profound impact of embracing our imperfections. As a coach, mentor, and women's spiritual empowerment leader, I have witnessed how our so-called flaws and missteps contain the seeds of transformation. By acknowledging and learning from these shadows, we unlock our true potential, emerging stronger and more empowered than ever before.

As we let go of our attachment to outcomes and surrender to the Universe's divine flow, we begin to see our imperfections as stepping stones to self-discovery and growth. Let us cherish our journey and the wisdom gained from both our triumphs and challenges. With each imperfection we embrace, we move closer to living authentically and wholeheartedly, trusting in the beauty of our perfectly imperfect selves.

Our imperfections are not shortcomings, but rather opportunities for transformation. By accepting and embracing our flaws, we unlock the potential for deep inner growth and understanding. As Wayne Dyer eloquently put it, by accepting our flaws, we can turn them into tools for self-discovery. These imperfections are not roadblocks on our journey but stepping stones leading us to our true selves.

Embracing our perfectly imperfect nature allows us to live authentically and in alignment with our deepest truths. It is our imperfections that add depth, richness, and beauty to life. By releasing the need for perfection and welcoming our flaws with open arms, we step into a space of empowerment and self-acceptance. Embrace your imperfections as beacons of light, guiding you toward a life of authenticity and fulfillment.

When we let our minds be consumed by beliefs of inherent flaw and perpetual imperfection, we inadvertently shrink our potential and dim the light of our true essence. Believing ourselves to be fundamentally flawed traps us in a sense of smallness and limitation, obscuring the beauty within our unique imperfections.

Instead of embracing our flaws as part of our authentic selves, we fall into the cycle of self-criticism and comparison, perpetuating negativity and self-doubt. By shifting our perspective, we can break free from this cycle and recognize the transformative power of our imperfections.

Internalizing these beliefs builds walls around our hearts and minds, closing off boundless possibilities. This self-imposed limitation stifles our creativity, dampens our spirit, and hinders our ability to fully express our potential. Fixating on our perceived flaws blocks the flow of self-love and acceptance, trapping us in a cycle of self-sabotage and diminished self-worth. Instead, by recognizing and embracing our imperfections, we can unlock our true potential and live authentically.

WORTHINESS

A former client of mine, Mary, carried the weight of inherited stories painting her as flawed and unworthy. Raised in an environment demanding perfection and harshly criticizing flaws, she internalized the belief that she was not enough. The dream of creating her own business, a passion that ignited her spirit, remained elusive as she hesitated, paralyzed by the fear of not measuring up to an unattainable standard. On her coaching intake form, she bravely wrote, *I never feel fulfilled, I pick fights with my husband, and I hate how short-tempered I am with my children.*

After a few sessions working through the Evolve & Evict process in my coaching program, she realized that lingering echoes of others' doubts had been driving her. These beliefs, planted long ago, had taken deep root and grown into tangled weeds, choking her true desires and leaving her trapped in a suffocating life.

During our journey of self-discovery and empowerment, Mary reclaimed her Authentic Self by addressing childhood wounds and confronting beliefs imposed by her parents. Together, we scripted and practiced a dialogue she would have with them. In a pivotal session, I role-played her parents while she expressed her inner child's (*Little Girl Big*) thoughts and feelings.

After weeks of sessions and one rehearsal, Mary started to feel more relaxed. She decided she wouldn't bury her desires anymore or live in fear of imperfection. She was tired of disappointing herself and no longer feared disappointing her parents.

I checked in with her between sessions to see how it went with her parents.. She texted me, *Jen, after voicing my needs out loud to you, something shifted within me. I felt free. I decided not to waste my breath on a discussion with my parents. My needs and boundaries are for me, not them. Whether they change or not doesn't matter to me anymore. I don't want to feel the fight anymore. I see my truth and I'm going to start making choices based on it.*

Mary reclaimed her voice and power, shedding limitations that hid her true self. With newfound clarity, she courageously transitioned from the corporate world to coaching women in narcissistic relationships.

Embracing her imperfections as catalysts for growth, she stepped into her purpose of believing in herself, which led her to supporting other women on a journey she knew well.

By embracing her flaws as part of her unique story, she found liberation and fulfillment in living authentically. As Mary emerged from self-doubt and societal pressures, she illuminated a path to authenticity, inspiring others to do the same.

It's crucial to acknowledge the harmful effects of fixating on perceived flaws and adopt a perspective that celebrates imperfection as part of our human experience. Shifting from self-criticism to self-compassion, as Mary did, supports personal growth, inner peace, and empowerment. When you break free from limitations and embrace imperfections, you become a guiding light on the journey to self-discovery and authenticity.

PATH TO PROGRESS

Embracing Imperfections: The Path to Authenticity and Growth:

- ☐ **Affirmation:** *"I live a perfectly imperfect life, embracing my flaws as tools for growth."*
- ☐ **Soul to Soul Message:** Your value lies in your imperfections. By sitting and embracing your flaws, you transform them into opportunities for growth and self-discovery.
- ☐ **Key Takeaways:** Highlight the importance of embracing imperfections as part of the human experience. Emphasize how accepting and learning from our flaws leads to authenticity and personal growth.

☐ **Action Step:** Reflect on a perceived flaw that has held you back. Write about how this imperfection can be viewed as a strength and a tool for personal growth.

If you liked this message, you may want to choose your journey to Evolve 1.6 or Expand 3.6.

Emerge Exploration

How can you embrace imperfections as assets for self-discovery and growth?

What steps can you take to release the pursuit of perfection and embrace your authentic imperfections for a more fulfilling life?

...

FORGIVENESS BRINGS PEACE

Atonement is your

salvation from fear,

anger, resentment and judgment.

Remember your truth:

You are LOVE.

2.7
LIFE HAPPENS FOR US, NOT TO US

Twenty-six years ago, my husband and I received the incredible news that I was pregnant with our first baby. The joy and excitement overwhelmed us as we embarked on a journey filled with new dreams for our growing family, and both of our families embraced us with wholehearted support, eagerly anticipating the arrival of their first grandchild.

But life took an unexpected turn, and our journey shifted from joy to sorrow. Sadly, our precious soul-baby stayed with me only briefly; early in my pregnancy, she returned to the angels. Twelve weeks was too short, and the loss left my husband and me heartbroken.

I couldn't understand why such pain had entered my life, yet, deep down, I felt it was safe to trust the unknown. So, I trusted. I cried. I grieved. And I cried more. Through my sorrow, I began to see how her soul would bless us with invaluable gifts that continued to reveal themselves over the next 26 years.

Through all the grief and uncertainty, life continued to throw challenges our way. It seemed as though everything happened in threes. First, my husband lost his job. Then, there was a grease fire in our apartment. Thankfully, it didn't cause much damage, but everything was covered in grease—from toothbrushes to dishes, rugs, and bedding—everything had to be cleaned with airplane degreaser. And then came the third blow—the most painful of them all—the loss of our baby.

I remember standing alone in the middle of our apartment, crying out, *Why, God, why?!* It was all too much to handle at once—his job, the fire, and now our baby. *How could this little soul we were so eager to welcome into the world change her mind? She didn't choose us. WHY?!*

It felt unbearable, yet in the midst of the pain, a voice inside whispered to my heart, *Life is unfolding for you. You are safe. You are loved.* Seriously? *How could this possibly be happening for my benefit?* My heart was shattered, and I felt utterly lost and alone.

In the weeks that followed, life seemed to settle into a rhythm of grief and survival. I focused on getting through each day, finding comfort in small, familiar routines. Then, something unexpected happened that would change the course of my life.

On a quiet Sunday afternoon, as I made my way back from taking out the trash, the familiar lyrics of *Amazing Grace* echoed repeatedly in my mind—*I was blind but now I see*. It struck me as odd to be singing that song out of the blue.

As I ascended the stairs to our apartment, tired from a day of mundane chores, I found my husband waiting for me at the door. His expression was solemn as he guided me to the living room and gently seated me on the couch. He began by saying he had something important to share.

Sensing the gravity in his gaze, confusion and panic washed over me as I braced myself for what was to come. What followed was a pivotal confession—he admitted to struggling with a drinking problem, and his admission shook me deeply.

I sat stunned, staring at him, thinking, *No, that can't be true. What are you saying? You must be mistaken.* His words left me in disbelief, and I was on the verge of interrupting to deny them. But then, as if in response to my internal turmoil, the song lyrics echoed in my mind once more: *I was blind but now I see.* I quieted myself, deciding to listen. To truly listen.

Matt poured out everything he had been wrestling with—the full weight of his addiction. The room seemed to spin around me as I tried to anchor myself into the couch while absorbing his words. It was his turn to sob, to grieve, his pain raw and unfiltered as he unloaded the burdens he had carried. Then, what he said next completely caught me off guard. Through his tears, Matt confessed, *It was my fault.*

Confused, I asked him what he meant.

The baby. I caused you to lose the baby, he responded, his voice breaking.

I was speechless. I couldn't comprehend how he could blame himself for the miscarriage. As I sat there, listening to him, it struck me just how deeply our loss had affected him. His anguish was profound, leading him to shoulder the blame. And in that guilt, he found the resolve to confront his addiction and begin his path to recovery.

Acknowledging his struggles with alcohol, Matt committed to sobriety—a decision that would redefine our lives. He entered rehab while I found solace in Al-Anon meetings. The following weeks were a whirlwind of change, with my own journey evolving alongside his recovery. Life began to reveal its threads of purpose as my husband embraced sobriety, a choice catalyzed by the aftermath of our loss.

His journey transformed everything. Slowly but surely, life began to fall into place in unexpected ways. Our pain and loss paved the way for a fresh start. Now, more than 25 years later, he continues to live a sober, healing life. Not a day passes without my deep gratitude for our baby, who chose a different path—for herself and for our future family.

That little soul paved the way for two more amazing souls to enter our lives: Jordan Matthew and Ashlyn Faith. The child who chose not to stay brought us more than we could have ever prayed for—a strong marriage, a beautiful son and daughter, and a life built on faith and self-trust. Embracing the truth that life happens for us, even in the toughest times, reveals gifts that are often waiting to be discovered.

EVERYTHING HAPPENS FOR A REASON

Before the miscarriage, I used to find comfort in the belief that everything happens for a reason, thinking there was purpose behind life's twists and turns. Over time, however, I began questioning this belief. It seemed I was constantly searching for explanations instead of fully living in the moment.

When facing challenges like missed opportunities, heartbreak, or the loss of our child, I would default to, *everything happens for a reason*. Yet, upon deeper reflection, I realized this mindset prevented me from fully processing my emotions and hindered my healing journey. Being fixated on the 'why' kept me from embracing the present moment and finding genuine peace and comfort.

Through a journey of self-discovery and growth, I came to understand that life isn't simply a series of predetermined events with specific reasons behind them. It's an ongoing journey of learning, where every experience offers an opportunity for personal development and deeper understanding. This realization shifted my perspective from *everything happens for a reason* to the profound truth that *life happens for us, not to us*.

LIFE HAPPENS FOR US, NOT TO US

Life happens for us, not to us marks a significant shift in perspective that can profoundly influence how we navigate life's journey. Instead of perceiving ourselves as passive recipients of random events, *Life happens for us* mindset encourages us to see each experience as a valuable opportunity for growth and evolution. It reminds us that we have an active role in how we interpret and respond to life's circumstances, empowering us to shape our own journey.

When we embrace the idea that life unfolds for our benefit, we empower ourselves to approach challenges with curiosity and openness. Instead of feeling like victims of fate, we become active participants in our own stories, capable of finding purpose and meaning even in the most trying times. This perspective encourages us to look beyond the surface of difficulties and setbacks, seeking the lessons and opportunities for personal development that lie beneath.

Life happens for us, not to us underscores our agency in shaping our reality. By acknowledging that we have the power to choose how we engage with life's ups and downs, we can cultivate resilience and inner strength. It prompts us to lean into discomfort and uncertainty, trusting that every experience, whether joyful or challenging, holds seeds of wisdom and insight that enrich our journey.

This mindset invites us to adopt a practice of gratitude and self-discovery, enabling us to approach life with purpose and clarity. It reminds us that, regardless of what life brings, we possess the capacity to transform adversity into opportunity and to discover meaning and fulfillment in the ebb and flow of existence.In essence, *life happens for us, not to us* invites us to view life not as a series of obstacles, but as a collection of experiences that shape a narrative of growth, resilience, and self-realization.

PATH TO PROGRESS

Life Happens for Us, Not to Us:

- ☐ **Affirmation:** *"I trust that life happens for me and embrace each experience as a gift for my growth."*
- ☐ **Soul to Soul Message:** Embrace the belief that life happens for you, not to you, and see every experience as an opportunity for growth and understanding.
- ☐ **Key Takeaways**: Highlight the importance of shifting perspective from being a passive recipient to an active participant in life's journey. Emphasize how each experience, whether positive or negative, offers lessons and opportunities for personal growth.
- ☐ **Action Step:** Reflect on a challenging experience in your life. Write about how it has contributed to your growth and what lessons you have learned from it.

If you liked this message, you may want to choose your journey to Evolve 1.7 or Expand 3.7.

Emerge Exploration
Where in your journey has life happened for you, not to you?

How does embracing this mindset empower you to navigate challenges?

· · ·

2.8
EMBRACE YOUR TRUE SELF: LESSONS FROM THE ARENA

Only accept opinions from those who are willing to join you in the arena.

At a young age, my son found his rhythm in basketball, just as my daughter discovered her passion for dance. Being their mom meant dividing my time between cheering at basketball games and being a dance mom at competitions. Navigating between scoring hoops and applauding pirouettes often made my head spin. I even called my son's uniform a 'costume' a few times. Despite the confusion, I recognized an intriguing parallel between their two worlds.

From the bleachers, where I tracked scores and times, a profound realization hit me. It was easy to spot missed passes and shots from a distance, to critique and point out what could have been done differently. Yet, as I watched parents in both settings—the basketball court and the dance stage—something became crystal clear: judgment and opinions flowed freely.

All bystanders had them. In basketball, voices echoed freely from the bleachers, with parents shouting advice and directions as if they were the coaches. At dance competitions, silence enveloped the audience, but the same whispers of critique lingered in the air.

Sitting among fellow parents, whether at home games or away, I noticed how effortless it was for them to voice opinions and judgments from the comfort of the bleachers, removed from the heat of the game. The cheers and jeers, the applause and disapproval—all felt distant from those in the arena, on the court, exposed and vulnerable.

As Brené Brown would say, we occupied the "cheap seats," far from the arena where the game of life unfolded. Reflecting on Roosevelt's timeless quote about the *Man in the Arena*, the poignant truth resonated deeply. The opinions we so readily offer from our seats in the stands hold little weight compared to the courage and vulnerability displayed by those on the frontlines, unshielded by distance or detachment.

In the dance of life, this distinction becomes even more evident. The voices from the bleachers fade against the backdrop of those daring to step onto the stage, take the shot, make the leap, and embrace vulnerability with unwavering courage. It is within the arena, where sweat mingles with passion and vulnerability intertwines with resilience, that true growth and authenticity thrive.

As we navigate life's challenges, it's crucial to value only the opinions from those willing to step into the arena with us. This guiding principle, in our exploration of self-discovery and growth, becomes a beacon of wisdom, gently nudging us to own our strengths and embrace our true selves. And in our quest to let go of unwanted opinions and embrace our own story, each experience, challenge, and detour becomes a vital piece of our personal growth. We learn to navigate the paths that lead us closer to our authentic selves.

The art of selective listening becomes crucial as we move towards deeper self-assurance. Imagine a colleague critiquing your work style or a fellow parent questioning your decisions. Are they qualified? Have they stepped into the arena with you, or are they sitting in the cheap seats? These moments highlight the importance of sifting through the noise and focusing on those who truly support your progress. This is where the skill of choosing whose feedback to value shines brightest.

DARE TO LEAD

Inspired by Brené Brown's *Dare to Lead*, consider cultivating a *Square Squad*—a circle of trusted allies whose insights and opinions you cherish. These individuals will serve as pillars of strength and guidance as you journey towards growth and authenticity.

To create your *Square Squad*, take a small piece of paper, like a post-it note or a tiny square torn from a notebook, and draw a one-inch by one-inch square. Keep this small token in your wallet or pocket as a tangible reminder of your support system.[2]

Within this square, write the names of those who embody trust and authenticity in your life. These are not people who simply tell you what you want to hear but those who are willing to be vulnerable with you and share their own struggles and failures. These individuals form your *Square Squad*, the ones you turn to for unwavering support and understanding.

Reflecting on my own journey, the *Dare to Lead* training from Brené Brown has been a cornerstone in both my personal and professional life. From the final chapters of my teaching career to my coaching endeavors and the way I conduct retreats and engage with clients, this program has been transformative.

---

[2] In Brené Brown's words, a Square Squad is a small group of people whose opinions of you truly matter. These are individuals who have earned the right to provide feedback and whose support you value deeply.

I highly recommend exploring the free resources available on the Brené Brown website: https://brenebrown.com/ under *Dare to Lead*. For those interested in delving deeper, the certification program offered by her team is a valuable opportunity. The course profoundly impacted me, sparking revelations about leadership dynamics and the essence of sharing power within a team.

During the training, one specific moment stands out to me. During one of the breakout sessions, my initial goal of enhancing my coaching and mentoring skills expanded into a profound shift in my teaching approach. The program highlighted the need for change within the education system, emphasizing the stark contrast between leading with power over others, and leading from a place of shared power.

True leadership honors the diverse contributions of the team members without feeling threatened by differing ideas. It supports curiosity and collaboration. This shift in perspective was pivotal for me, transforming how I approached both teaching and leadership.

As you immerse yourself in this book and its transformative journey, a stronger, more authentic version of yourself will emerge. You will discern who to include in your *Square Squad*, valuing those who uplift and support your growth. Through this process, you will recognize that the opinions of those in the cheap seats hold less weight as you embrace your true essence and confidently embody your Authentic Self.

PATH TO PROGRESS

Embrace Your True Self: Lessons from the Arena:

> ☐ **Affirmation:** *"I trust my true self and embrace the lessons from the arena."*

- ☐ **Soul to Soul Message:** Only accept opinions from those who are willing to join you in the arena.
- ☐ **Key Takeaways:** Emphasize the importance of valuing opinions from those who support and understand your journey. Highlight the concept of the *Square Squad* and the power of selective listening.
- ☐ **Action Step:** Reflect on the people whose opinions you value. Create your own *Square Squad* by writing down the names of those who embody trust and authenticity in your life. Keep this list as a reminder of your support system.

If you liked this message, you may want to choose your journey to Evolve 1.8 or Expand 3.8.

Emerge Exploration

When have you let the opinions of people outside your trusted circle affect your decisions or how you see yourself?

Who would you include in your Square Squad—those trusted allies who truly support and uplift you with honest insights and unwavering encouragement?

• • •

**The Universe will follow your lead.
It will never push or pry you open.**

Your power lies in surrendering to the flow of your life.

AND SO IT IS.

2.9

THE TRANSFORMATIVE POWER OF MOMENTUM

Momentum will carry you farther than any dream.

As I opened my eyes on the morning of my 8th birthday, I couldn't contain my excitement. But that excitement quickly turned to disappointment and sadness when it seemed my parents had forgotten about my special day. Still in my pajamas, no one wished me a *Happy Birthday*. Instead, my dad asked me to get the shovel from the garage and pick up the dog poop in the backyard before the day got too hot.

I felt incredibly sad and angry (my grown-up self understands the anger, but back then my *Little Girl Big* only felt safe to feel sad). I couldn't understand why I had to be on poop patrol on my birthday. But being the 'good girl' I was back then, I stuffed my sadness, put on my gaucho pants and angel-winged shirt, and headed out to the garage.

I hated the garage. It smelled musty, and there was always a spider or two waiting to welcome me. As I turned the handle and pushed open the door to the garage, tears brimmed in my eyes. I truly thought my birthday had been forgotten. But to my surprise, the shovel I expected to see in the corner was replaced by a magnificent Huffy banana-seat bike, adorned with pink and white flowers and streamers cascading from the handles. I was NOT on poop patrol after all; I was being celebrated for the big girl I was becoming.

I wasted no time running back to my parents, who were waiting outside with the Polaroid camera to capture the moment. I hugged them, showered them with kisses, and asked them to teach me how to ride.

With eager anticipation, I embarked on my first ride down our bumpy sidewalk. Its uneven stones and pebbles challenged my balance and determination. But with my dad cheering me on and holding the back of the banana seat, I pressed down on the pedals. The cool air brushed against my face as I teetered and wobbled, feeling both fear and exhilaration with every push. Each rotation of the wheels brought a growing sense of steadiness and growth.

The familiarity of uncertainty and the thrill of moving ahead despite the shaky start resonated deeply within me. Little did I know those early rides on my banana seat bike would mirror my life's journey to come - a blend of resilience, discovery, and the transformative power of momentum.

In much the same way, momentum, propelling us beyond mere dreams and aspirations, depends on taking action. It's about pressing forward with unwavering dedication, fueled by passion and purpose that illuminate our path. Just like my bike ride, where the uneven terrain smoothed out with each push, life beckons us to stride with courage and conviction, trusting that momentum will carry us further than mere dreaming or passive observation.

In those moments, I learned that progress isn't always smooth or predictable. It's about embracing the bumps and trusting the process. Each wobble, each moment of uncertainty, becomes a step towards growth and transformation. And so, I pedaled on, finding balance and joy in the journey, knowing that with every push forward, I was moving closer to my true self.

I can't say I never fell off that Huffy. It was less about falling off and more about getting back on. Each tumble I took off my pink banana seat bike, each scraped knee my mother tended to with a loving touch and a mercurochrome smile, taught me a lesson in resilience and staying present. It wasn't always the uneven stones under my wheels that caused the falls—it was the moments of distraction, the twirl of thoughts taking me away. The truth of my falls mirrors life's journey, where thoughts of regret often linger around the paths not explored and the dreams left untouched.

In the adventure of embracing a heart-centered life, we are drawn toward uncharted paths, not by abandoned dreams, but by the hidden potentials waiting to be brought to light. The dreams that linger in our thoughts can't come alive just by thinking about them. They need us to take a leap, to step into the unknown, guided by our choice to follow love, not fear.

In the journey of life, where fear and love silently dance, many of us hold back, muffling the whispers of our true desires in the haze of uncertainty. Yet, with each brave move we make, with every spark of momentum from our actions, our dreams find the nurturing soil to grow and thrive. Each movement forward, each leap of faith, paints a portrait of bravery, endurance, and unyielding resolve and helps us see we are capable of bringing our dreams to life.

Failure, once seen as a shadow of weakness and shame, now emerges as a guiding light of wisdom and growth. When I was teaching I displayed a sign in my 8th-grade classroom that boldly declared, **FAIL: First Attempt In Learning**, serving as a source of empowerment for my students. It was a daily reminder that mistakes are stepping stones paving the path to growth and wisdom.

As we navigate everyday life, we realize the importance of action over mere thoughts. Staying safe by staying small, doesn't cut it any longer.

Each stumble and success, each moment of exploration and connection, lead us toward turning dreams into reality. It's the continuous push forward, the relentless pursuit of momentum, that breathes life into our aspirations. By staying the course and not letting external opinions sway us, we become the architects of our own happiness.

The law of attraction, often misunderstood as a mental exercise, finds its essence in action and intent. Thinking is just the beginning; making things happen involves taking action, exploring, connecting with others, seeking guidance, and gaining knowledge. In the end, it's the determination to keep moving forward that transforms our dreams into living, breathing parts of our story, shaping who we are and where we're headed.

PATH TO PROGRESS

The Transformative Power of Momentum

- **Affirmation:** *"I embrace the power of momentum and let it carry me beyond my dreams."*
- **Soul to Soul Message:** Momentum will carry you farther than any dream.
- **Key Takeaways:** Emphasize the importance of taking action and embracing progress, even when it's not smooth or predictable. Highlight how momentum builds resilience and fosters growth.
- **Action Step:** Identify one dream or goal you have been hesitant to pursue. Take a concrete step toward it, no matter how small, and observe how momentum begins to build.

If you liked this message, you may want to choose your journey to Evolve 1.9 or Expand 3.9.

Emerge Exploration

When doubt or fear arises, what small step can you take today to move closer to your dream?

Think of a time when others' opinions or fears influenced your choices. Consider how those influences were more about them than you.

...

2.10

THE POWER OF ABUNDANCE AND GRATITUDE

Freedom comes from embracing what you have.

Abundance extends beyond material wealth, encompassing the intangible gifts that truly enrich our lives—love, compassion, creativity, and meaningful experiences. It encourages us to adopt a mindset of plenty, seeing the endless opportunities around us. How can we imagine having more if we can't appreciate what we already have? According to the universal law of attraction, we attract more of what we are, not what we want. The more grateful we feel, the more abundance we attract, and the freer we become.

Reflection and appreciation plant the seeds of freedom and abundance, but it's action that nurtures those seeds and helps them grow. While embracing gratitude and recognizing the richness of our lives is a powerful beginning, true liberation comes when we transform those feelings into purposeful action. Just as a gentle breeze sets a sail in motion, our actions create the momentum that carries us beyond the shores of dreams.

By taking thoughtful steps and staying committed, we turn gratitude into a powerful force that moves us toward true freedom. Each action shows our progress on the path to abundance and joy. This journey to deeper freedom starts with facing our inner struggles and making peace with our past. When we shift our focus from simply enduring hardship to celebrating our strength, we open the door to a life full of gratitude and abundance. Letting go of the pain frees us to embrace new possibilities and guides us toward a future filled with fulfillment and peace.

GATEWAY TO AUTHENTIC FREEDOM

Gratitude and abundance are gateways to authentic freedom. True freedom comes from appreciating what we already have, cherishing the little moments, simple joys, and blessings that we often take for granted.

When we pause to notice these small pleasures and the relationships that nourish us, we awaken to the richness of our lives. Gratitude shifts our perspective from what's lacking to what's present, creating contentment and fulfillment in the moment.

True freedom isn't found in external validation or possessions. Instead, it grows from embracing gratitude and abundance, which help us feel more whole and connected to the world around us. This mindset deepens the richness of our inner lives and builds a strong foundation for self-discovery and growth.

In the hustle of chasing our dreams, we sometimes overlook what we already have. While inspired action and releasing past pains support our growth, balancing this with a recognition of our current blessings is the key to inner richness and authentic liberation. Abundance isn't just about material wealth; it's about embracing the love, kindness, and experiences that shape our existence. By focusing on appreciation rather than scarcity, we unlock a world full of endless possibilities.

BRIDGING THE GAP

The road to freedom isn't cluttered with accolades or unattainable dreams. It's a humble journey of gratitude for the present moment and the beauty it brings. It's about shedding the weight of fear to step into the brilliance of our potential.

Too often, we find ourselves ensnared by the chains of our desires, held captive by the pursuit of external wants.While setting goals and pursuing aspirations can drive success, the fundamental truth remains clear: we unknowingly confine our happiness to material possessions, whether it be money, a romantic partner, the latest trend, or any sought-after possession.

This belief ties us to an unending pursuit of temporary sources of joy, driving us to conform to societal norms in a constant search for fulfillment. In other words, we become controlled by our desires, trapped in the gap between what we have and what we believe will make us happy once we attain it.

True happiness remains elusive until we realize it cannot be tied to external acquisitions or societal standards. Genuine contentment thrives when we resonate with the frequencies of abundance and appreciation, regardless of our external circumstances.

It is not the size of our bank account that determines life's richness, but rather the state of gratitude and satisfaction in which we reside. For those immersed in abundance, the realm of possibility expands without bounds, bridging the gap between current reality and envisioned dreams. When we break free from societal expectations and the myth that we'll never be satisfied, we will start to experience a profound shift toward true fulfillment.

When we awaken to abundance and appreciation, it lights up a path to a profound frequency of joy, love, and freedom. It goes beyond the usual story of what happiness means, replacing it with a model of intentional living. True freedom emerges not as a final destination but as an ongoing journey, offering endless possibilities for self-realization.

Freedom is a dance of the heart. It's in the tender moments of gratitude, the acts of abundance, and the spark of manifestation that we discover the profound beauty of freedom. Freedom springs from within, blooming from embracing the wealth of our inner world. It transforms the typical story of happiness, opening up a new way of living where we choose and act with intention, empowering us to create our own journey to true fulfillment.

PATH TO PROGRESS

The Power of Abundance and Gratitude:

- ☐ **Affirmation:** *"Freedom comes from embracing what I have."*
- ☐ **Soul to Soul Message**: Embrace abundance beyond material wealth and focus on love, compassion, creativity, and experiences.
- ☐ **Key Takeaways:** Highlight the importance of shifting focus from scarcity to appreciation, understanding that true happiness and freedom come from within.
- ☐ **Action Step:** Reflect on the non-material aspects of your life that bring you joy and fulfillment. Write down ways you can cultivate a mindset of gratitude and abundance.

If you liked this message, you may want to choose your journey to Evolve 1.10 or Expand 3.10.

Emerge Exploration

Where in your life do you notice yourself imprisoned by the pursuit of achievement rather than savoring the beauty of appreciation?

How can you break free from chasing success and instead focus on appreciating the abundance in your life?

...

Affirmation of Inner Freedom

Freedom springs from within me,

blooming through gratitude,

abundance, and intentional action.

I embrace the wealth of my inner world,

choosing and creating

my own journey to true fulfillment.

2.11

REGRET AS YOUR GPS: COURSE CORRECTION

*Regret is not a lesson. It's a misunderstanding
in thinking your experience was a mistake.*

Regret, often viewed negatively, carries the weight of past choices and actions. It can act as both an anchor, grounding us and a barrier, holding us back beneath turbulent waters. In our journey of emerging self-discovery, we confront the limiting beliefs and societal imprints that have shaped our perception.

As we explore this journey further, we begin to see regret in a new light. No longer a place of sorrow and remembrance, regret transforms into a guiding compass, leading us toward growth and transformation. It becomes a hidden gem—an opportunity to rewrite the story, moving beyond the simple categorization of right and wrong. As we surface for a breath in this phase of emergence, we are tasked with redefining our understanding of regret.

When regret is embraced with courage and clarity, it becomes a catalyst for change. Rather than dwelling in the shadows of past missteps, we harness its power to create momentum and propel us forward. It invites us to rewrite our stories, let go of the past, and rediscover our authentic selves.

Releasing regret honors our evolution, acknowledging that every stumble and detour has crafted the path to our present selves. We navigate the terrain of gratitude and self-compassion, recognizing that our past actions were borne of the wisdom and understanding available to us at the time. We had to be where we were to be where we are now.

In the embrace of gratitude, regret transforms into a source of insight. It illuminates the contrast between our past and present, guiding us toward conscious choices and authentic self-expression. Through this transformative process, regret ceases to be a burden and emerges as a gift—a teacher of resilience and compassion.

FROM REMORSE TO WISDOM

With this insight, we can turn regret from a shroud of remorse into a source of wisdom. In this section of emergence, we rise above the waves of self-doubt and shame, revealing the power of rewriting our inner narratives. Regret, viewed through the lens of growth and acceptance, becomes a tool for deeper healing and development.

I've personally felt this shift in my own life. Eight years ago, during a coaching retreat in Kentucky, I had an experience that reshaped my journey forever. Meeting my first life coach, I was skeptical about the need for guidance, but that moment changed everything.

I literally thought, *A life coach? Who needs a coach to live life?* But just minutes into the coaching exercise, I found my answer. At that time, I was not someone who easily showed my emotions, so I was mortified when tears welled up during the exercise, exposing a flood of buried regrets and deep sadness. I found myself unable to contain the emotions I had long suppressed. I was shocked by the depth of my sadness, especially since we were asked to recall a happy memory.

The memory surfaced quickly: a flash of my four-year-old son playing at the beach. It was a wonderful memory, so why did it make me feel so sad? In a vulnerable instant, I could not hold back my confusion.

Through streams of tears and shallow breaths, I tried not to blubber as I blurted out, *Why is a happy memory making me cry?* The question lingered as I wrestled with my emotions—*Why was I swimming in a sea of sadness?*

I don't remember the exact question she followed up with, but I do remember the clarity it brought. Already in tears, I was suddenly overwhelmed by a deeper flood of regret and sadness. My sorrow stemmed from the belief that I had missed precious opportunities to cherish my son's childhood innocence. A pang of shame hit me as I realized how I had overlooked the simple beauty of his young life. The fear of judgment and the pressure to mold him into a 'good boy' had clouded my joy during those fleeting years of his childhood.

The life coach approached me and guided me further into the experience, where I recognized even more regret- if that was even possible. I believed I had stolen my son's joy by turning everything into a lesson instead of being present for his moments of fun, laughter, and silliness. I realized I had been so busy trying to mold him that I missed the fun he brought to each moment in my life. Blinded by my own insecurities and fears of falling short as a parent, I believed I had stolen his joy.

This realization marked a turning point in my journey. As the retreat came to an end, I felt a deep sense of clarity. The insights I gained weren't just revelations to ponder—they were calls to action. I returned home with three truths guiding me forward. *First*, I knew I needed to dive deeper into the story I was telling myself about my son. *Second*, I realized it was time to seek out a life coach of my own. *And finally*, with unwavering certainty, I understood that becoming a life coach was part of my path.

Upon returning home, I took the first step and hired a life coach. With his guidance, I began making incredible shifts, releasing many of the limiting beliefs that had held me back. However, even with this progress, it took time before I was truly ready to sacrifice my suffering and free myself from the story I had created around my son's stolen joy.

It wasn't until a recent visit to my parents' home, while watching old family videos, that my regret was truly challenged. As we laughed and reminisced, I began to see my son's childhood in a new light. His carefree laughter and playful antics painted a picture of joy and love I feared I had stifled. Watching him giggle with infectious joy on the screen, I realized he didn't seem to be missing anything. Could my story have been wrong?

In that moment, I had the opportunity to evolve, evict limiting beliefs, and emerge anew. In a vulnerable moment, I turned to my adult son and shared my regrets, apologizing for being too strict and robbing him of his carefree spirit.

To my utter surprise, he responded with disbelief, affirming that his childhood had been filled with happiness and love—nothing like the story regret had been telling me. His simple words shattered the self-imposed narrative I had created. In that moment, I realized I had been carrying a burden of guilt that was never mine to bear. Embracing his truth negated the limiting beliefs I had built in my head and affirmed the reality. I released the weight of past regrets and chose to emerge from the shadows of self-doubt.

With his perspective, I found the courage to let go of the pain that had held me captive for so long. Free from the shackles of self-doubt and fear, I chose to emerge from the shadows, releasing beliefs that no longer served me. Regret, once a heavy burden, transformed into a gentle guide—no longer something to fear, but a GPS for growth and course correction. And this is a tool we all have. Regret can become a powerful teacher, helping us realign with our true path. Instead of letting it weigh you down, try seeing it as an opportunity for reflection and course correction. Embracing regret with love and understanding can guide you toward healing, deeper self-awareness, and a life lived more authentically.

PATH TO PROGRESS

Transforming Regret into Growth:

- ☐ **Affirmation:** *"I transform regret into wisdom and growth."*
- ☐ **Soul to Soul Message:** Regret is not a lesson; it's a misunderstanding in thinking your experience was a mistake.
- ☐ **Key Takeaways:** Emphasize the importance of viewing regret as an opportunity for growth rather than a source of shame. Highlight the transformation of regret into a guiding compass for self-discovery and empowerment.
- ☐ **Action Step:** Reflect on a regret you have been holding onto. Write about how you can reframe it as a source of wisdom and growth.

If you liked this message, you may want to choose your journey to Evolve 1.11 or Expand 3.11.

Emerge Exploration

How has regret been keeping you from living an authentic life?

What would it feel like to release regret to receive peace and joy?

YOU ARE NEVER CHAINED TO A CHOICE.

SURRENDER YOUR FEAR AND CHOOSE AGAIN.

2.12
THE POWER OF HEALING: EMERGE AS YOUR AUTHENTIC SELF

You hold the light to heal the world.
By healing yourself you heal the Earth.

We've been taught that life is full of lessons and hardships and that we need to struggle through them. But I challenge this belief. Where did it come from? I am not saying we don't experience struggle, challenges, and burdens at times. We do. Yet, there is a profound difference between what we feel and what we have been taught to believe. The mind is a powerful tool for growth, but it can also be a barrier to healing if we cling to false beliefs and old narratives.

We came here to experience all that life has to offer, but somewhere along the way, we misunderstood the assignment—like one of those Instagram Reels where everyone's in on the joke but us. Life isn't about ticking off boxes or chasing perfection. It's about embracing the messiness, the joy, and all the lessons along the way. This misunderstanding highlights why we need to engage in the healing process, with the very first step being awareness and evolution.

That's where evolving comes in. Evolving is about dissecting, examining, and getting curious about these beliefs. When we recognize where we have been gifted—yes, gifted—these beliefs, we can then decide what we want to continue carrying with us and what we need to release.. This process guides us back to our personal truth, our sovereignty.

And the truth is, this life is a giant playground—a beautiful, magical, sometimes challenging, sometimes painful contrast of experiences. It is a gift for us to explore and embrace. When we remember that *life happens for us, not to us*, we stay out of the victim mentality.

We begin to connect the dots, like a constellation of repeated patterns and choices we have made. We clear our vision, and we see the truth. We take responsibility for our choices, and in doing so, we gain immense power—power within ourselves, not power over others.

You are the light that holds the power to heal the world. By healing your soul, you heal the Earth. Each of us, no matter who we are, is always interconnected. We are never alone.

After evolving and emerging, we come up for air and see the world through a new sense of sight, free from others' limiting beliefs. Embracing this newfound perspective, we begin to see that regret is not a lesson but our personal GPS. Regret is simply a guide, helping us navigate our past experiences in a neutral map.

It provides us with information without the weight of shame, guilt, or negativity. This realization allows us to view our past choices as experiences rather than mistakes, freeing us from the burden of regret and empowering us to fully step into our power.

The Emerge section builds upon the foundations laid in the Evolve section, where we explored the concept of *light attracts light*. Understanding that what we put out into the world comes back to us was the first step in recognizing our power. Now, as we emerge, we see how this attraction works on a larger scale. Our healing radiates outward, impacting not only ourselves but also the entire world.

This inner power allows us to see our choices clearly, to choose again, and to understand that everything we do comes from our legacy of light—our soul's spark. Recognizing this truth helps us see others in theirs. Some may be confused or living in chaos, but when we are grounded in our own truth and connected to our Authentic Self, we no longer feel the need to overpower or fix them. Our purpose in this lifetime has never been to preach or convert. Each person has their own journey, and not everyone will walk alongside us. There's no need to judge or condemn their choices—judgment of others often reflects the judgment we hold toward ourselves.

As we heal, we deepen our connection to our inner light—our true, authentic essence. In this growth, we learn to honor the unique paths of others. Holding space means being present without judgment, offering support while respecting the individuality of each person's journey.

Our healing radiates outward, like throwing a pebble into a lake and watching the ripples spread far and wide. Each ripple touches the entire pond, just as our energy impacts the world around us. No matter our nationality, gender, race, or country, we are all interconnected through collective energy.

Energy is everything. We can feel it, read it, and sense it in ways that go beyond words and expressions. You've experienced this when you walked into a room and immediately sensed whether the atmosphere was welcoming or tense.

This awareness of energy is not new. Science addresses it as *The Law of Conservation of Energy*, which teaches us that energy cannot be created or destroyed, only transformed. Our purpose is to transform this energy and use it for healing and growth.

By healing yourself, you remember your purpose. You are the golden cog in the wheel of life, essential to the collective. Your healing impacts countless lives, often in ways you may never see. We often seek immediate understanding and proof, but true knowing comes from experiencing. When you do this work, you reach a level where proof is no longer necessary. You simply know. And the *knowing* is everything.

You hold the light to heal the world. By healing yourself, you share in the healing of every creature, every tree, and the Earth itself. There is no separation. Separation is the greatest pain we know; it is the belief that we are not connected. This belief leads to feelings of isolation and exclusion. But by evolving, emerging, and expanding, we recognize our interconnectedness. We remember that we are never alone.

Above all, know this: you are the center of the wheel, with all spokes connected to you. You hold the light to heal yourself, and in doing so, you heal the world. Embrace your role as the host of your life, release the need to control every outcome, and know that life is always happening for you. Your light and your journey are the catalysts for profound change. You are that powerful!

PATH TO PROGRESS

The Power of Healing: Emerge as Your Authentic Self

- ☐ **Affirmation:** *"I hold the light to heal the world. By healing myself, I heal the Earth."*
- ☐ **Soul to Soul Message:** Embrace the belief that healing yourself contributes to healing the world. Recognize the interconnectedness of all beings and the impact of your personal growth on the collective.

- ☐ **Key Takeaways:** Understand that life is a journey of learning and growth. Emphasize the difference between what we feel and what we have been taught to believe. Highlight the importance of evolving, examining beliefs, and transforming energy for healing and growth.
- ☐ **Action Step:** Reflect on a limiting belief you have held onto. Write about how this belief has shaped your experiences and how you can shift it to embrace your true self and contribute to collective healing.

If you liked this message, you may want to choose your journey to Evolve 1.12 or Expand 3.12.

Emerge Exploration

How does your personal healing influence those around you? Reflect on a time when your growth inspired someone else.

What daily practice can you adopt to nurture your light and contribute to the collective healing of the world?

. . .

Angel Prayer for Healing and Authenticity

Archangel Raphael, Divine Healer,

We call upon your radiant presence to guide us on our journey of self-discovery. Help us to release the fear and limiting beliefs that keep us small. Illuminate the truth of our divine magnificence, reminding us that we hold the power to heal the world.

Grant us the strength to embrace our authentic selves, to evolve beyond the shadows and emerge into the light of our true essence. Let us see that by healing our own souls, we contribute to the healing of the Earth.

May we recognize the interconnectedness of all beings, knowing that we are never alone. Teach us to transform the energy within and around us, using it for growth and profound change. Help us to hold space for others on their journeys, respecting the diverse paths we each travel.

Fill our hearts with gratitude, abundance, and the spark of manifestation. Show us that true happiness and freedom come from within, empowering us to create our own journey to fulfillment.

As we heal, may our light radiate outward, touching lives far and wide. Let our energy ripple through the world, bringing love, peace, and joy to all.

Archangel Raphael, we ask for your guidance to live in alignment with our authentic truth. Help us to see that we are the center of the wheel of life, with the power to heal ourselves and, in doing so, heal the world.

We thank you for your eternal presence and the profound love you share. May we always remember our role in the collective, and embrace the journey with open hearts and unwavering faith.

Amen.

SECTION III

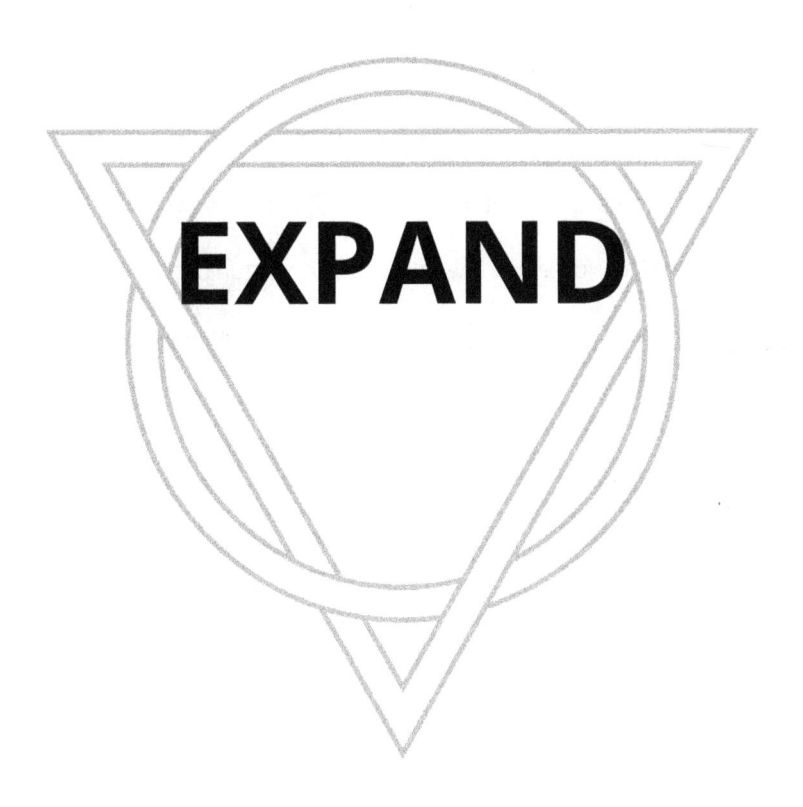

EXPAND

A PRAYER FOR EXPANSION

Beloved Council of Light,

Guide my hands, my heart, my mouth, and my feet.

When I start clinging, remind me to surrender.

When I ignore you, speak up louder than before.

When I make it about me, help me get out of my own way.

When I am fearful, let me see my fears as opportunities to expand.

Thank you for working through me throughout my day.

And so it is.

~Rebecca Campbell
Light is the New Black

3.1

Choosing Courage over Comfort

Brave is not asking anyone what brave looks like.
"Daring greatly is being brave and afraid every minute
of the day at the exact same time."
~Brene Brown

Expanding your authenticity starts with living your life without waiting for permission, showing others they can do the same. *To achieve this, you must choose courage over comfort, or as Brené Brown says, dare greatly.* As she puts it, *To love ourselves and support each other in the process of becoming real is perhaps the greatest single act of daring greatly.*

Many of us adopt the fears of our families and friends. Though their opinions and advice often come from a loving place, they carry the weight of their own limiting beliefs, which keep them playing small.

Fear and love run neck and neck in their power over us. If a thought shows up in the energy of fear, it has likely woven itself deep into your physical body. Most people don't recognize the warning signs that they are making decisions from a place of fear, not love. They are also unaware that fear gives them cues about where pain is being stored in their body.

Most times, I feel my fear in my gut, specifically in the solar plexus. I literally find myself holding my stomach when a fearful thought comes up. I literally find myself holding my gut when a fearful thought comes up. This is a new realization for me; I used to think my fearful thoughts were housed in my head until my Reiki practice helped me understand otherwise. I dug deep and emerged from my shadow work with the realization that fear had been living rent-free in my gut, not my head. My fearful thoughts had been showing up as undigested toxins in my body, manifesting as gluten intolerance, dairy intolerance, and finally, a sick gallbladder.

As I mentioned earlier, the body keeps score. For me, fear was definitely winning while my physical health was losing. My body was sending me cues that fear was hiding in my gut, but I kept ignoring them. I ignored them for so long that the only way they could finally get my attention was through my gallbladder attacking my body. It wasn't a shock when the ER doctor informed me that my gallbladder needed to be removed because it was bursting with sludge. SLUDGE! Seriously, eww! And yes, sludge is actually a medical term.

I felt a deep sense of truth and gratitude in the doctor's message. Truth because, when I connected all the dots—or rather, sludge stones—I realized I had been living in fear for most of my life. And gratitude because I wasn't facing a more serious health condition.

The night I made my midnight run to the ER, I was in the midst of a profound spiritual upleveling. What most would see as a gallbladder attack, I recognized as a return to consciousness that brought me to my knees. My family was shocked to hear I needed to have it removed because they saw how clean I ate—no gluten, no dairy, limited sugar. But I wasn't surprised at all. My body had been absorbing all the fear I was experiencing, storing it in my gallbladder to keep me safe.

I had close friends advise me on how I could heal my gallbladder homeopathically, but my gut spoke to me in love and told me a different story. I knew without needing proof that it was time to remove my gallbladder. It was time to face and release the fear it had been protecting me from. I knew it was time to trust myself, to trust my gut, to be brave, and to stop asking everyone else what brave looked like.

I shifted into a healthier state of mind, body, and spirit by choosing courage over comfort. My body knew it no longer needed to store my fear. It trusted me to take over.

It trusted me to choose from love.
It trusted me to remove the shields I once needed to keep me safe.
It trusted me to no longer be afraid of my power.
It trusted me to reenter the flow of my life.
It trusted myself to step back into my power and choose to be brave.

What is your body asking of you? Is it asking for trust? Is it urging you to be brave, without needing anyone else's definition of bravery?

Choosing to be brave means not asking for anyone else's permission. It means aligning with your authentic beliefs and releasing the beliefs taught by others that no longer serve you. Choosing courage over comfort is defining bravery for yourself.

PATH TO PROGRESS

Choosing Courage Over Comfort:

- ☐ **Affirmation:** *"I choose courage over comfort, trusting my inner strength and wisdom."*
- ☐ **Soul to Soul Message:** Embrace the power of courage by listening to your inner voice and choosing actions that align with your Authentic Self. True bravery comes from within, and it doesn't seek external validation. By daring greatly, you inspire others to do the same.

- ☐ **Key Takeaways**: Emphasize the importance of recognizing where fear resides in your body and understanding how it affects your decisions. Highlight the need to trust your intuition and release limiting beliefs passed down from others. Reinforce the idea that courage is about being true to yourself, not seeking approval from others.
- ☐ **Action Step:** Reflect on a recent decision where you chose comfort over courage. Identify the fears that influenced your choice and where you felt them in your body. Write down one action you will take this week that aligns with your authentic self, even if it feels uncomfortable. Practice mindfulness to tune into your body's signals, and notice how it responds when you act from a place of courage.

If you liked this message, you may want to choose your journey to Evolve 1.1 or Emerge 2.1.

Expand Exploration
Where does your body hold fear?

Where in your life can you be brave and choose courage over comfort?

• • •

**Your growth comes through choosing courage over comfort.
Curiosity, creativity, and courage connect you with your Divine Power.**

AND SO IT IS.

3.2

CLAIMING YOUR HAPPINESS
You shift, they shift.
*"Do the best you can until you know better.
Then when you know better, do better."*
~Maya Angelou

If only _____ (name) would change this or stop doing that, then I would be happy. Has this thought ever crossed your mind? I used to live with it replaying in my head for years.

Looking back, I realize I had mastered the art of pointing out everything others needed to change for me to feel worthy, happy, and at peace. In fact, I spent the better part of my first year working with my life coach repeating, *If they would just believe in me, stop saying..., start saying..., stop doing..., start doing..., then I could be happy.*

My coach has the patience of a saint because he never gave me advice or told me what he already knew: *If I continued to seek my self-worth and happiness in the opinions and actions of others, I would never find it.* Instead, he waited, listened, and asked all the right questions for me to realize I held the key within me to create my own happiness regardless of the circumstances around me.

Before this self-discovery, I left the door wide open for depression and anxiety to make their grand entrance time and time again. This does not mean I believe I caused these feelings, nor am I against medicine for the support it can offer in navigating depression and anxiety. In fact,

I am grateful for how medical intervention helped me get back on track. Still, I had reached a point where I felt I could manage without it if I had the right tools.

I should add that I gave myself permission to continue with antidepressants if needed—without judging myself as a failure. This was an important agreement as I moved forward on my journey.

Until I began to learn otherwise, I had no idea that I held the power to create pockets of happiness independent of others' moods. I didn't realize I could be supportive and loving without absorbing the emotions of those around me. I was autonomous in myself, and my happiness didn't depend on theirs.

For a long time, as a people-pleaser, I believed that if someone wasn't happy, it was my job to fix them and make them happy. If I did my job right, we'd both be happy. Later, I realized this was how the narcissist in me, the empath, was showing up. Empaths feel so deeply that we want to control how others feel in order to avoid their negative emotions. This realization was a major eye-opener for me.

I've come to understand I have the power to choose my mood, my happiness, and the direction of my life. With this knowledge, I made the conscious choice to take back the power I had been giving away. And so can you.

Before that *aha* moment, I had been allowing others to dictate my moods, my reactions, and my joy. It never occurred to me that I was the permission slip I had been looking for. I have the power to choose to be happy without the approval of others. This was an amazing discovery.

Previously, I had been letting others dictate my level of happiness. I was happy when my parents were happy. I was happy when my teachers were happy. I was happy when my husband was happy. And I was only as happy as my happiest child.

As Maya Angelou said, *Do the best you can until you know better. Then when you know better, do better.* Well, now I know better and I can do better for myself and expand my understanding in order to do better for those around me.

I now understand that I am the CEO of my emotions. I am in control of what happens within me. I choose to shift the thoughts that connect to the emotions I feel. I choose not to judge my emotions. I choose to remember they are ALL worthy of being felt. I choose to shift when I am ready. I choose not to be tofu and absorb the flavors and emotions of others .P.S. This last one is easy—Tofu has never been my jam.

YOU SHIFT, THEY SHIFT

With this shift, I discovered something even more cramazing[3]! When we shift our thoughts, energy, and emotions, we allow others to shift as well. Not by telling them what to do or how to act. Not by controlling them. We allow them to shift by showing them our authentic and grounded emotions and by giving them the freedom to choose for themselves. To love them enough to let them live their story. We no longer attach our happiness to their emotions.

Free will gives them the power to shift and match our vibration or stay rooted in what they are feeling. There is no judgment. There is no forcing. There is no right or wrong. There is only unconditional love which honors that which we feel.

---

[3] Linda Burgess, a Spiritual Mentor and beautiful soul sister, shared this word with me many years ago after a gorgeous sound bath healing she performed for the women at my retreat. She combined the words crazy + amazing to form CRAMAZING! This is the word I reach for when something feels so deliciously amazing in my soul.

By owning your level of happiness and not forcing others to give it to you, you expand your reach and your vibration to show others what it looks like to live an authentic life.

PATH TO PROGRESS

Claiming Your Happiness:

- ☐ **Affirmation:** *"I am the creator of my happiness, and I choose joy independent of others' actions."*
- ☐ **Soul to Soul Message:** Embrace the realization that your happiness is not dependent on the actions or opinions of others. Recognize your power to create your own joy and peace, regardless of external circumstances. By shifting your own energy and mindset, you can positively influence those around you without trying to control them.
- ☐ **Key Takeaways:** Highlight the importance of understanding that happiness comes from within and is not dictated by others. Emphasize the role of personal responsibility in choosing thoughts and emotions. Introduce the concept of transmuting negative energy into positive, and how your inner shift can inspire those around you.
- ☐ **Action Step:** Reflect on a recent situation where you felt your happiness was dependent on someone else's actions. Identify the beliefs and thoughts that contributed to this feeling. Write down one positive thought or affirmation that supports your autonomy in creating happiness. Practice this affirmation daily, especially in moments when you feel influenced by others' emotions. Observe how your shift in energy affects your interactions and the environment around you.

If you liked this message, you may want to choose your journey to Evolve 1.2 or Emerge 2.2.

Expand Exploration

Where could you be more authentic by freeing yourself from absorbing others' emotions? Spend some time today noticing if you rely on others for your own happiness.

Don't force any changes—just observe and gather information to decide if a shift is needed.

...

3.3

THE POWER OF ASKING QUESTIONS

Get curious.
Ask more questions and you will receive more insight.

The way to solve a problem is not to look for solutions but rather to ask more questions. I saw how your eyebrows furrowed as you read that line, and I know what you're thinking: *She's lost it,* but I haven't. Not about this, anyway.

As a middle school teacher of twenty-seven years, I can tell you the most valuable learning comes from asking questions, not just finding answers. When we focus solely on answers, we miss the valuable experiences that come from exploring the questions.

The goal of finding an answer is to feel a sense of ease and relief from the problem you are experiencing. But here's the issue—most of us put feelings of peace, ease, comfort, or joy on hold until we get an answer or find a solution to our problem. By doing this, we slow the momentum of our life, and our intention of feeling good moves farther out of reach.

When will I find the love of my life?
Is this the right job for me?
What is my purpose in life?
Why do I struggle with finances?

The problem does not lie in the unknown answers. The true issue is that we get so hyper-focused on the answer that we hit pause on living life, while we wait for it to arrive. We mistakenly believe the answer will bring us the happiness we seek.

It's very similar to "You shift, they shift." Before understanding the truth that you hold the power to create pockets of your own happiness separate from the situation, you must recognize where you have been giving away your power to others: their actions, their words, their choices, their moods. Through the journey of this book, now you know more. And when you know more, you do better. You know your moods, words, and choices alchemize not only your energy but the energy of those around you[4].

With your newly gained wisdom, you are breaking through inherited beliefs and replacing them with your own truths. Give yourself kudos and gratitude for the work you are doing to remember and return to your Authentic Self.

As you continue this path of self-discovery, remember that the journey is more important than the destination. And this, my friend, is where it gets exciting! On this journey you are breaking through self-limiting beliefs while also expanding yourself to move past your fears.

This will enable you to ask more questions without putting your life on hold, waiting for answers to find happiness. You will find your flow and continue to move forward through curiosity, asking questions that will expand you to be open to new possibilities, experiences, and a deeper understanding of yourself.

---

[4] In spiritual terms, to **alchemize** means to transform or transmute energies, emotions, or experiences into higher states of being or understanding. It's the process of turning challenges into opportunities for growth and enlightenment.

One of the greatest gifts of returning to your Authentic Self is the freedom to find happiness without depending on outcomes. Doesn't that sound absolutely *cramazing (page 146)*!? No more waiting or attaching your happiness to an answer. You are too powerful to live as a victim to uncertainty. Your happiness lies in embracing curiosity and asking true questions.

I will always be a teacher, whether within the four walls of a classroom or sharing with you here in this book. This is a model to help you shift from getting stuck searching for answers to reclaiming your power through the curiosity of asking powerful questions.

MODEL MOMENT

LIMITING QUESTION Question attached to answer:	POWERFUL QUESTION Question to shift thinking:
When will I find the love of my life?	How can I show myself more love? Where am I not romancing myself in life? What does a loving gesture look like for me?
Is this the right job for me?	What lights me up? Where do I find joy in life? What am I learning from my current job? Example: communication, patience, compassion, forgiveness.
What is my purpose in life?	Am I living and working from a place of love? When do I feel most fulfilled in life?

	What themes do I see in my life? Example: helping people, communicating, supporting, creating.
Why do I struggle with finances?	Am I able to recognize abundance in my life? What do I currently have that I'm grateful for? What are my opinions about people with money?

Can you sense the journey the questions on the right will lead you on? By shifting your focus away from questions like *When will I find the love of my life?*, you stop fixating on what's missing and reclaim your power. You're no longer a victim, tying your happiness to a single answer. Instead, you become curious. The more curious you become, the more aware you are of your beliefs. This awareness allows for subtle shifts, helping you live in flow and attract more happiness into your life.

PATH TO PROGRESS

The Power of Asking Questions:

- ☐ **Affirmation:** *"I embrace curiosity and let it lead me to growth."*
- ☐ **Soul to Soul Message:** Ask more questions, and you will receive more insight.
- ☐ **Key Takeaways:** Focus on questions, not just answers. Understand that the journey to solutions lies in asking the right questions rather than solely seeking answers. Detach from outcomes. Learn to find peace and happiness in the process of inquiry, without attaching your well-being to the answers. Empower through curiosity. Use curiosity to shift your thinking, breaking through self-limiting beliefs and expanding your perspective.

☐ **Action Step:** Reflect on a current challenge in your life. Write down the questions you are seeking answers to, then reframe them into powerful, open-ended questions. For example, instead of asking, *"When will I find the love of my life?"* ask, *"How can I show myself more love?"* Practice this reframing daily and observe how it shifts your mindset and opens up new possibilities.

If you liked this message, you may want to choose your journey to Evolve 1.3 or Emerge 2.3.

Expand Exploration

Make a running list of limiting questions you have been asking about your life. Use the model above to rewrite the limiting questions in a powerful way.

Where are you pausing your life to find an answer before you take action?

3.4

THE POWER OF BELONGING
Create a tribe and call them in.

The ego tends to get a bad rap. The truth is, the ego thinks she's doing us a favor by protecting us from rejection, so she discourages us from putting ourselves out there and taking risks to make new connections. The ego doesn't do well with bravery. She doesn't want us to risk more dismissal and exclusion.

Think of it this way—the ego is like a helicopter parent who wants the best for her child. She means well by being protective but ends up hurting more than helping. She smothers you, preventing your light from expanding and keeping you from being truly seen.

When the ego hovers over our choices, she cuts us off from knowing our authentic selves and finding the tribe where we truly belong—a tribe where we don't have to change ourselves to fit in. Without a deep understanding and love for ourselves, we end up searching for a tribe to force ourselves into, a place where we have to fake it till we make it. And that NEVER feels right.

What do we do when our ego throws a temper tantrum? Often, we get caught up in her lies and fear-based stories, running for cover and hiding. Some of us hide so well and for so long that we become invisible, even to ourselves. Over time, we forget our authentic selves.

Here's a powerful truth our ego hides from us: **rejection isn't personal**. The circles we long to fit into aren't our true tribe if we have to change who we are. To fit in, we often shrink ourselves, sacrificing our truth and essence to meet others' expectations.

Belonging is not synonymous with fitting in. To belong is to feel safe and empowered to connect with those who share similar interests and beliefs. It's where vulnerable, messy, and powerful conversations can happen. Here, respect for our differences and a willingness to get it wrong are more important than the comfort of silently fitting in.

Belonging is where we stand in our power and invite other outliers to join us. There's no need to whittle away our authenticity or play small to be chosen. When you choose yourself, you become a magnet for others to find you. Connection within creates connection throughout.

When we become aware of the lies our ego has been speaking, we remember we have the freedom to choose again. We can choose to release the false stories and reconnect with our Authentic Self. This is when we begin to embrace vulnerability as our superpower.

Vulnerability is courage wrapped in skin. It allows us to see our worth and expand into the world as our Authentic Self. Rejection protects us from circles that desire conformity, giving us clarity of sight through our hearts. This is how we see where we truly belong.

When I began working with my life coach, I opened up to him about the deep sadness in my soul from never feeling like I fit in. Not in Catholic school, public school, college, as a teacher, or with other mothers. I felt like I was always on the outside, caught in a never-ending game of Farmer in the Dell. Always being held at arm's length outside the circle, never being called into the center.

I had friends, but they didn't really know me because I was hiding my Authentic Self. Wearing a mask to fit in only left me feeling even more disconnected.

How my coach responded to my feelings of exclusion changed my life. He was quiet for a moment, then looked at me and asked, *Why do you keep looking in the same direction? It's such a small circle you're trying to fit in. Why don't you turn around and begin to explore the rest of the world? Look for a new circle.*

What? Turn around? Could it truly be that simple?

Yes, it was that simple for me, and it can be for you too. Who doesn't want to make life simpler? I lived in 'the hard' for far too many years—the part where I felt alone, sad, and rejected. A lot of that time was spent in victimhood. After spending so much time in the shadows, I figured, how hard could it be to live in the light? My light.

Why don't you look for a new circle?

No thank you. I was done searching for a tribe to fit in with. Been there, done that. It was time to expand my light and create my own damn circle—a tribe where we belong to ourselves and each other.

It was time to release the fear of being seen and judged, especially since people didn't even know the real me because I had been hiding my Authentic Self for so long. It was time to expand myself big enough for my tribe to find me.

To see me. To know me. To love me as my Authentic Self.

The change will happen for you too when you start recognizing the voice of the ego. By quieting the ego, you can hear the whispers of your spirit. Your Authentic Self isn't a red flag to keep people away but rather your superpower, your red cape, inviting them in.

Putting on my red cape allowed me to expand and create the *Miracle Minded Woman* Facebook Community, retreats, oracle cards, a book, and a tribe. Being seen is what allowed you to find me here, in these pages.

When we stop hiding, we can finally be found—and that goes for you, too. When you embrace your true self and step into your light, the right people, opportunities, and experiences will find their way to you.

PATH TO PROGRESS

Embracing Your Authentic Self: The Power of Belonging:

- ☐ **Affirmation:** *"I embrace my Authentic Self and call in my tribe."*
- ☐ **Soul to Soul Message:** True belonging is about being seen for who you truly are. Release the fear of rejection and connect with others who appreciate your authentic self.
- ☐ **Key Takeaways:** Understand the ego. Recognize that the ego, like a helicopter parent, tries to protect you from rejection but ends up preventing you from connecting with your true tribe. Reframe rejection. Remember that rejection is not personal but a sign that you were not in the right circle. Embrace vulnerability. See vulnerability as your superpower, allowing you to connect with your Authentic Self and attract those who truly belong in your life.
- ☐ **Action Step:** Reflect on moments in your life where you felt you had to hide your true self to fit in. Write down these experiences and the emotions they stirred in you. Then, turn the page and list ways you can embrace your Authentic Self and call in your tribe. Consider joining groups or communities that align with your interests and values, and commit to showing up as your true self.

If you liked this message, you may want to choose your journey to Evolve 1.4 or Emerge 2.4.

Expand Exploration

What fears are you willing to surrender in order to be seen?

How will you expand and call in your tribe?

...

The Power of Belonging

Create a tribe and call them in,

where your light can shine without fear.

The ego means well but hovers too close,

shielding us from bravery,

smothering our true selves.

She whispers lies of unworthiness,

making us believe we must fit in,

to circles never meant for us.

Belonging is not fitting in,

it's standing in your power,

 inviting others to join,

without shrinking to be chosen.

Rejection is protection,

leading us toward our true tribe,

where we belong to ourselves,

and others who see our light.

Turn around, explore the world,

create your own circle,

expand your light, be seen,

for when we stop hiding,

we can finally be found.

3.5

Navigating the Journey of the Empath
How Narcissism Shows Up in the Empath

*"In a world of armored hearts, vulnerability
is the bravest armor we can wear."*
~Brené Brown

For empaths, awareness is our North Star, guiding us through the rollercoaster of emotions we navigate. It's a realm where empathy reigns supreme, and we navigate the delicate balance between light and shadow. At the heart of this journey lie two opposing forces: narcissism and empathy.

Personally, I've always seen myself on the side of empathy. I viewed narcissism as my sworn enemy, the force that disrupted my peace. I invested a lot of energy guarding against narcissists and their draining ways. But as I dug deeper, I discovered something profound: the empath's power doesn't come from building walls against narcissism. Instead, it grows from understanding, accepting, and rising above it.

I was shaken to the core when I learned that I, too, could share some traits of the narcissist. *What? Me? No, not me! I was the good one.* I believed narcissists to be bad, evil—not that I was judging or anything (insert sarcasm and major eye-roll here). I struggled to embrace the idea that I might have traces of narcissism within me.

Although the idea repelled me, it also intrigued me. If there's one thing I've learned through my journey of the soul, it's to lean into the very situation or idea that triggers me. It's to get curious and ask more questions because our triggers are the GPS to deeper understanding and enlightenment. Using my triggered narcissist map, I was able to uncover the intricate dance between narcissism and the empath.

Those of us who identify as empaths find ourselves deeply attuned to the emotions of others, drawn to the intricate nuances that paint the human experience. Our compassionate nature supports a natural inclination to offer support, understanding, and healing to those around us. Yet, nestled within the depth of empathy lies the potential for narcissistic manifestations.

Sometimes our ego has a hidden agenda we are not aware of. Undermining the truth of our empathic nature, our ego may be silently and sneakily seeking validation and recognition from others through external reassurance. In other words, your ego may be using your goodness and nice actions as a ruse while she looks for validation to confirm your worth and goodness.

Jen is such a good person. Jennifer is the go-to girl for everything we need. Isn't she just the best!?

Who doesn't like to receive praise? Praise fed my soul. Or so I thought. The truth is, it was really feeding my ego. If you've ever felt resentful after offering to do something nice for someone, it was most likely because your actions and intentions were not aligned. Your Authentic Self didn't plan on offering because you already knew you were stretched thin and couldn't take on any more.

Your Authentic Self has beautiful boundaries and didn't plan on crossing them. But your Authentic Self didn't get the memo or the invite to do the talking. Instead, your *Little Girl Big* (ego) offered to be nice and volunteered anyway, leaving you feeling very frustrated and resentful.

Your ego pulls the strings more than you know - until now. She does not make decisions from a heart-centered place. She makes them from fear - past memories, stories and insecurities. The ego's intention is to make sure you are not left out. She will make choices to ensure you are seen and praised as nice, rather than focusing on genuinely performing a kind act. Niceness is ego-centered, disconnected, and seeking recognition. This is how traits of a narcissist can surface within the empath.

I told you it was sneaky.

Part of the reason it's so sneaky is because the ego hangs out at the unconscious playground. She is the unhealed inner child: *Little Girl Big*. And she wants to be accepted, liked, appreciated, and revered for her goodness. She wants to be told she is a good girl.

Did you know that ninety-five percent of our choices are made in the unconscious—the very place our inner child lives? It's true. So, don't be too hard on yourself if you're just now realizing that your ego has hijacked your well-intentioned, kind, and empathetic choices. You are not alone. This is why it's so important to engage in inner work, as you are doing with this book.

You cannot alter what you are not aware of. Awareness is the key to unlocking the door of transformation and transcendence away from narcissistic tendencies. The empath is highly sensitive and doesn't want to feel rejected, so they will continue to show up and attempt to fix a situation and offer assistance to avoid negative feelings of sadness, rejection, or fear. Although their actions may be nice and supportive to others, if they are working from the place of avoiding feeling rejected, they won't be aligned with love.

As empaths gain a deeper understanding of themselves, the entanglements of narcissism will begin to release their grip on the heart. With each step toward self-awareness and self-compassion, they empower themselves to release the need for external validation, finding peace in the richness of their inner light. In this radiant space, they illuminate the way for others, guiding with empathy, compassion, authenticity, and a spirit of expansion.

In the sections to follow, we will explore the many facets of the empath's journey, discovering the transformative power of empathy when it converges with wisdom and self-love. By weaving these elements together, we pave the way for a harmonious dance where authenticity and strength converge to create a profound connection with both ourselves and the world around us.

PATH TO PROGRESS

How Narcissism Shows Up in the Empath:

- ☐ **Affirmation:** *"I embrace my empathy with awareness and strength from my inner light."*
- ☐ **Soul to Soul Message:** Embracing your empathy with awareness transforms narcissistic tendencies into authentic, heart-centered actions.
- ☐ **Key Takeaways:** Recognize that the ego often seeks external validation under the guise of empathy. Learn to distinguish between ego-driven niceness and genuine kindness. Understand that most choices come from unconscious drives. Shift from seeking external validation to finding strength in your inner light and Authentic Self.
- ☐ **Action Step:** Reflect on moments of resentment after offering help. Journal to determine if your actions were driven by a

need for validation or genuine kindness. Identify patterns where ego influences your decisions. Commit to one change this week, choosing heart-centered kindness over seeking recognition.

If you liked this message, you may want to choose your journey to Evolve 1.5 or Emerge 2.5.

Expand Exploration

Where has your unhealed inner child hijacked your good deeds in order to receive praise for being good?

How can you make peace with her and show her more love?

...

3.6

THE RIPPLE EFFECT

By Healing your Heart you Heal the Collective Heart

"When you heal your heart, you are healing the world. As you heal your own wounds, you are contributing to the collective healing."
~Rebecca Campbell

As you continue on the journey of expansion, remember this truth: by healing your heart, you are not only nurturing your own soul but also impacting the collective consciousness. Every act of self-love, forgiveness, and healing reverberates beyond the confines of your being, weaving threads of light and healing through the interconnected web of humanity.

In this space of growth and evolution, the power of vulnerability and authenticity becomes your guiding light. Embracing your imperfections and honoring your journey, you pave the way for profound transformation within yourself and the world around you. Let your healing radiate outwards, creating ripples of love and healing that transcend boundaries and unite us in a shared journey of growth and awakening.

Imagine your heart as a drop in a vast ocean, connected to every other drop around you. When you heal your own heart, you're not just making yourself feel better—you're sending out positive vibes that reach out and touch the hearts of everyone around you. It's like smiling at a stranger on the street and brightening their day, or lending a listening ear to a friend in need and making them feel supported and understood. By taking care of your own emotional well-being and spreading love and kindness, you contribute to an invisible web of positive energy that uplifts us all. It's about realizing that we're all in this together and that a little act of self-love can go a long way in creating a world where we all feel connected and supported.

Recall a time when someone entered your life like a burst of sunshine, their positivity contagious and uplifting. Their joy likely brightened your day, lifted your spirits, and brought a smile to your face. Now, think about a moment when someone's negativity or bad mood seeped into your state of mind, casting a shadow over your outlook. Their energy may have left you feeling drained or disheartened, affecting your well-being in a tangible way.

These experiences remind us of the interconnectedness of our emotions. By reflecting on how others' vibes have influenced your mood, you begin to see the ripple effect of emotional energy and its profound impact on our collective well-being. In these moments of shared energy and resonance, the truth of healing your heart to heal the collective heart becomes vividly clear.

Rebecca Campbell's quote, *When you heal your heart, you are healing the world. As you heal your own wounds, you are contributing to the collective*, speaks to a powerful truth on our journey towards inner healing and growth.

By taking care of ourselves and showing compassion towards our imperfections, we not only improve our own lives but also spread positivity and healing to others. True happiness comes from within, not relying on others' approval or happiness. Focusing on self-love and acceptance creates a ripple effect of love and kindness that uplifts and inspires everyone around us.

This journey of self-discovery involves balancing self-care with nurturing healthy relationships, without losing our sense of self. Embracing our own healing and growth transforms our lives and contributes to a more compassionate world.

WHEN I BLESS YOU, I BLESS ME

After my experience with my superintendent and principal (*Evolve 1.6*), I continued my healing and self-discovery journey in my professional life. I embarked on a journey of forgiveness and self-realization, aiming to be true to myself, authentic, and living from a place of integrity. Through past shadows, I embraced my inner light and navigated a path of growth.

In my last two years as a Special Education Teacher and Consulting Teacher of the Deaf, I immersed myself in deep healing with the support of a spiritual therapist and my life coach. This led to significant shifts, including a deliberate decision to reduce my inner circle of friends.

Through my healing, I uncovered old traumas and embraced the truth that life happens for us, not to us. Despite the challenges and triggers—especially with my superintendent—I persevered and returned to a neutral space where those triggers no longer held power over me.

After two years of dedicated healing work, I made the conscious choice to retire early from teaching, not as an escape, but as a testament to my commitment to personal growth and healing. By the time I bid farewell to that chapter of my professional life, I could face my superintendent with a heart free of palpitations and a mind clear of anxiety.

Each day, as I drove to school, I offered blessings to him, extending compassion and releasing any ties that bound me. With my departure, a ripple effect occurred—my principal moved to a new district, the superintendent followed suit a year later, and even my Special Education Supervisor embarked on a new journey. Through healing myself, I unknowingly facilitated healing within the collective, releasing old wounds and paving the way for new beginnings.

In a poignant conversation with my principal before his departure, we shared a moment of understanding—the realization that healing oneself ultimately extends to healing the collective. As compassion flowed between us, I found the courage to speak from a place of truth and authenticity, words that had been veiled during previous times of hurt and turmoil. I conveyed to him the depth of his impact, recognizing his inherent qualities of excellence and kindness, and acknowledging that this district was not harnessing the full breadth of his potential.

I urged him to release the chains of pain and resistance, and to sever ties with the past in order to step into his new chapter unencumbered. For him to shine brightly in his next position in a new district, it was imperative to leave behind any shadows of blame or resentment, to embrace a fresh start with clarity and purpose. Through this truthful conversation and mutual understanding, everything changed—he found a new direction, a school embraced his talents, and his heart was filled with the joy of following his true calling.

This is the essence of healing—the journey within ourselves that radiates outward, touching lives and illuminating paths. By tending to our own wounds and embracing our true essence, we not only find solace and renewal but also become guiding lights for those around us. As we heal ourselves, we inadvertently heal the collective, creating a ripple effect of growth, understanding, and profound transformation.

PATH TO PROGRESS

The Ripple Effect of Healing:

- ☐ **Affirmation:** *"By healing my heart, I contribute to the collective healing."*
- ☐ **Soul to Soul Message:** Embrace the truth that healing your heart nurtures not only your soul but also the collective consciousness. Each act of self-love, forgiveness, and healing sends out ripples of positivity, uniting us in a shared journey of growth and awakening.
- ☐ **Key Takeaways**: Recognize Interconnectedness: Understand that your healing impacts the collective, creating a web of positive energy. Embrace Vulnerability: Honor your journey by embracing imperfections and supporting authentic connections. Transformative Power: Realize that your personal healing contributes to a compassionate and harmonious world.
- ☐ **Action Step:** Reflect on moments when someone else's energy affected your mood, both positively and negatively. Journal about these experiences and how they influenced your well-being. Commit to a daily practice of self-love and forgiveness, acknowledging that each act of healing within yourself contributes to the collective heart. Practice spreading positive energy through small acts of kindness and observe the ripple effect it creates.

If you liked this message, you may want to choose your journey to Evolve 1.6 or Emerge 2.6.

Expand Exploration

How can I embody compassion and forgiveness towards others, realizing that healing myself contributes to the healing of the collective?

In what ways can I release past pain and resentments, allowing myself to step into a new chapter with clarity, purpose, and authenticity?

...

Blessing of the Ripple

May you heal your heart and become the ripple, spreading love and compassion from the depths of your şoul.

In each act of self-love and moment of grace, may you touch the interconnected web of humanity, reaching lives far and wide.

As a drop in the vast ocean, may your light and soul merge with others, creating waves of transformation and unity.

Through your healing journey, may you become the water, flowing with purpose, illuminating paths, and making the world whole.

3.7

SUBTLE MIRACLES IN EVERYDAY LIFE
Miracles are shifts in perceptions.
"When you change the way you look at things, the things you look at change."
~Wayne Dyer

In everyday existence, miracles often reveal themselves subtly. These fleeting moments hold the key to unlocking the extraordinary within the ordinary. Wayne Dyer's wisdom reminds us that changing how we see the world can transform the world we see.

As we explore miracles, we witness the connection between healing our hearts and nurturing the collective soul. The healing ripple from within us transcends the individual *Self*, creating unity and compassion. Embracing the miraculous within, we become deeply connected to the radiant healing light of wholeness.

Life unfolds with purpose and intent. Every experience carries a hidden message waiting to be revealed. By remembering *life happens for us, not to us*, we empower ourselves to embrace each moment as a stepping stone toward growth and enlightenment. This perspective invites us to dance in harmony with the Universe, aligning our hearts and minds with the cosmic symphony.

Growing up, I thought miracles were only talked about in church. Attending Catholic school, I learned of miracles as big and amazing events. But as I matured, I began to see miracles in the ordinary moments of everyday life. Miracles, I discovered, are found in simple acts of grace, like choosing kindness over resentment or forgiveness over holding a grudge. They exist in the small details of life that often go unnoticed. Shifting how we see a situation, being open to listening, and choosing understanding over getting upset are all part of experiencing everyday miracles.

I learned that miracles aren't just about big, extraordinary events but about the choices we make each day. By seeing things differently, listening with an open heart, and considering that everyone has a story, we open ourselves up to a world of miracles. The simple act of being open, understanding, and kind even in challenging times, can create a ripple effect of positive change.

Embracing this shift in perception extends its impact beyond ourselves. This practice of openness and understanding radiates into the lives of our loved ones, our communities, and the world at large.

PARENTS

Imagine a parent who sees the miracles in the mundane, guiding their children with grace and empathy. By modeling compassion and openness, they instill in their children the value of seeing the world through understanding and kindness. This nurturing environment supports connection and empathy in the next generation, creating a ripple effect that extends far into the future.

FRIENDS

Among friends and spouses, viewing each moment as a potential miracle creates deeper connections and meaningful relationships. By listening with empathy, communicating openly, and choosing understanding over judgment, individuals create spaces of trust and authenticity where bonds are strengthened and hearts are opened.

TEACHERS

In a classroom setting, a teacher who practices listening with an open heart and seeing the beauty in everyday moments cultivates a safe and supportive space for students to thrive. By embracing curiosity and understanding, they inspire students to approach learning with enthusiasm and empathy. These students, in turn, carry forward lessons of openness and compassion into their interactions, creating a classroom culture rooted in respect and understanding.

As a dedicated teacher with 27 years of experience, including the last 20 as a Special Education Teacher focusing on language and literature for eighth graders, I navigated a realm often considered challenging. Yet, despite its complexities, the eighth grade held a special place in my heart. I discovered that eighth-grade students were far more open and receptive than society often gives them credit for.

By approaching my role with authenticity and a genuine willingness to connect with each student, I was able to break through their barriers as they navigated their own phases of questioning authority, self-discovery, and search for belonging.

Eighth grade became an instrumental year of growth and transformation, not just for the students but for myself. Each September I embarked on a journey of mindset work, laying a foundation of trust and understanding before fully engaging in academics. I needed to walk the talk, signaling to my students that I was there to support and uplift them in remembering their worth and potential.

BEING A STUDENT OF MIRACLES

While the word miracle may not have been directly mentioned in my classroom, the essence of believing in the extraordinary was present in every interaction. I have always known that by nurturing my heart, I could initiate healing and growth within the collective spirit of my class.

This belief extends beyond the classroom, envisioning a ripple effect as my students went out into the world, each carrying the potential to inspire and create positive change. Each day, as I stepped into the classroom, I carried the faith that miracles were brewing, waiting to unfurl in the most unexpected ways.

Witnessing miracles in my classroom, from once-silent students finding their voices, to acts of vulnerability and genuine connection, I saw the transformative power of belief and understanding. I cherished the moments when students opened their hearts, shared their innermost thoughts and creations, and celebrated each other's successes. These were the moments where the ordinary turned extraordinary and where the mundane revealed its hidden treasures of connection.

SOPHIA

In one particularly transformative moment, a student we'll call Sophia started the school year hiding behind a long curtain of bangs, shielding herself from being seen and connecting with others. Despite her silent demeanor and reluctance to engage, her intellect and creativity shone through her work, hinting at a depth waiting to be seen.

One day, noticing Sophia's quiet passion for drawing, I reached out and shared a bit about my own love for art from years ago. This simple exchange of openness and curiosity sparked a miraculous shift within her—a gradual unveiling of her talents, her voice, and her worthiness to be seen.

Day by day, through sharing her drawings and embracing her newfound courage, Sophia emerged from the shadows, revealing a radiant spirit eager to connect, engage, and inspire those around her.

This journey of self-discovery and empowerment echoed the transformative power of embracing one's true Self and allowing miracles to blossom in unexpected ways.

Where do you find miracles in your life? In quiet moments of reflection, small gestures of kindness, or synchronicities that defy explanation? Embrace the shift in perception, for therein lies the myriad of miracles weaving through your existence. Just as I witnessed miracles in my classroom, may you recognize the miracles that grace your path and illuminate your journey toward a deeper understanding of Self and others.

PATH TO PROGRESS

The Subtle Miracles of Everyday Life:

- **Affirmation**: *"I am open to seeing the miracles in everyday moments and embrace the shifts in my perceptions."*
- **Soul to Soul Message:** Embrace the subtle miracles that surround you in everyday life. By shifting your perspective, you unlock the extraordinary within the ordinary, transforming your world and contributing to the collective healing.
- **Key Takeaways:** Recognize the Power of Perception: Understand that changing the way you see things can transform your experiences. Embrace Everyday Miracles: See miracles in simple acts of kindness, forgiveness, and understanding. Impact the Collective: Realize that your individual healing creates ripples that positively affect others.
- **Action Step:** Reflect on a recent experience where you felt challenged or frustrated. Journal about how shifting your perspective could reveal a miracle within that moment. Practice finding and appreciating the subtle miracles each day,

whether it's in a kind gesture,or a new understanding. Notice how this practice influences your overall sense of well-being.

If you liked this message, you may want to choose your journey to Evolve 1.7 or Emerge 2.7.

Expand Exploration
Where do you see the essence of miracles unfolding in your life today?

How can embracing a shift in perception open new pathways to self-discovery and empowerment in your journey?

...

3.8
THE POWER OF IMAGINATION
Your imagination is your truth.
"Imagination is the spark that ignites the fire of creation."
~Richard Wagner

I used to love stretching out on the grass, losing myself in the ever-shifting shapes of the clouds. It was like nature's own art show, with animals, castles, and secret worlds unfolding in the sky. As adults, we often label such things as imaginary, dismissing them as silly pastimes that exist only in a child's mind. But it is so much more.

Growing up, I often found myself lost in imagined conversations, voicing truths I couldn't express out loud. These whispered dialogues in front of the mirror were my way of connecting with my innermost feelings, serving as a lifeline to my true self. Over time, the notion that imaginary meant fake or unreal began to unravel, revealing a deeper layer of authenticity beneath the surface.

Unfortunately, for a while, I joined the masses in believing that the imaginary was fake. In my role as an eighth-grade teacher, I often reinforced this belief. I'd share a memory trick to help students differentiate between fiction and reality: *Think of the 'F' in 'fiction' and 'fake,'* I'd say. *Fiction isn't real. It's imaginary—fake.*

This mindset traps us, dismissing the power of our imagination as mere flights of fancy. Little did I realize back then that imagination is the very essence of our truth, the genesis of all that we create in our lives. Every structure, idea, dream—they all have their roots in the boundless realm of imagination.

We underestimate the profound impact of our imaginative thoughts by confining them to the realm of make-believe. Yet, the truth lies in the fact that our beliefs, the very fabric of our reality, are often shaped by fear—fear of judgment, fear of rejection, fear of not measuring up.

Take a look around you, whether you're reading the words on this page or listening to the audio version. Whether you're in a classroom, an office, a cozy living room, or a bustling kitchen, every object and detail around you was birthed from a spark of imagination.

What if we dared to challenge these limiting beliefs? What if we embraced our true, authentic selves without fear of external judgment? Imagine the possibilities that would unfold if we tapped into the wellspring of our imagination, creating a space where our truths could thrive and blossom.

Richard Wagner once remarked, *Imagination is the spark that ignites the fire of creation*. In those words, I found a profound truth that resonated with my experiences. The boundary between what is deemed *real* and *imaginary* blurred, revealing the transformative power within our thoughts and imaginings.

It's a shift in perception, a miracle waiting to be embraced—the realization that our beliefs are not truths but merely thoughts we've held onto and repeated for far too long.

Imagination holds the key to rewriting our narratives and crafting a life that reflects our deepest desires and visions. Let go of the fear that shackles you to outdated beliefs and embrace the liberating power of imagination. You have the ability to shape your reality.

Step into the arena of your imagination, where judgment holds no power and creation knows no bounds. Harness the magic of imagination to sculpt a life that is authentically yours, unbound by the chains of fear and doubt.

In the journey of self-discovery and growth, we stumble upon a fundamental truth: **miracles are not far-off events but mere shifts in how we perceive life.** Our imagination finds its home in these miraculous shifts, reshaping our view of what is true and possible.

Here's a key insight to help you tap into your most Authentic Self: **be selective with opinions.** Only those willing to step into the arena with you, ready to dig deep and get real, deserve a seat at your table. In this dance of holding space for your own truths while filtering out the noise, you open up to a world of expansion.

By weaving together the magic of your imagination with the strength of your convictions, you carve out a path that is uniquely yours, brimming with authenticity and boundless potential.

PATH TO PROGRESS

Embracing the Power of Imagination:

- ☐ **Affirmation:** *"I embrace my imagination as a powerful tool for creating my authentic truth."*
- ☐ **Soul to Soul Message:** Imagination is the spark that ignites the fire of creation. By embracing your imaginative thoughts, you connect with your innermost truths and unlock boundless possibilities.
- ☐ **Key Takeaways:** Recognize the Power of Imagination: Understand that imagination is the essence of creation and the foundation of our truths. Challenge Limiting Beliefs: Let go

of fears and outdated beliefs that confine your imagination. Embrace Authenticity: Allow your imaginative thoughts to guide you in creating a life that resonates with your true self.

- **Action Step:** Reflect on a limiting belief that has held you back. Write down how you can reframe this belief using your imagination to create a new, empowering narrative. Practice visualizing this new narrative daily, and notice how it influences your thoughts, actions, and overall perspective on life.

If you liked this message, you may want to choose your journey to Evolve 1.8 or Emerge 2.8.

Expand Exploration

How can you harness the power of your imagination to redefine your perceptions of what is possible in your life?

How can you stay true to your Authentic Self while balancing your own beliefs with the opinions of others, deciding which to accept and which to let go?

• • •

"I am enough of an artist to draw freely upon my imagination. Imagination is more important than knowledge. Knowledge is limited. Imagination encircles the world."

~Albert Einstein

3.9

AUTHENTIC PEACE AND POWER

Balance is the marriage of power and peace.

"You expand into the capacity to hold your own worth while being in relationship with another, without the need to control or dominate. The other becomes an ally and co-creator in life's journey rather than a threat to one's identity or beliefs."
~Alexandra Pope & Sjanie Hugo Wurlizter, Wise Power

The essence of authentic power and peace weaves through every interaction and moment, shaping the core of our being. This truth became evident during the 2020 lockdown, a time marked by unprecedented division among friends, families, and nations. Unlike age-old conflicts rooted in religious beliefs, this time it was the question of sovereignty over one's body that divided communities like never before.

During this time, a realization emerged in me: the fear-driven need to impose beliefs on others, regardless of origin or support, stemmed not from a place of balance or peace but from deep-seated anxiety, insecurity, and fear. As the lockdown continued, families were torn apart by the relentless pursuit of external validation, sacrificing their inner equilibrium and freedom. With growing concerns about health and mortality, the battle to change minds and assert dominance left many feeling lost and alone.

In the midst of this chaos, finding the union of power and peace within oneself became a beacon of hope and resilience. Authentic power, nurtured from within, expands to bring a profound sense of balance and inner knowing. It provides a steady, unshakeable foundation. This balance isn't about asserting superiority or righteousness but about standing firmly in your truth, grounded in the wisdom of both heart and mind. This inner alignment, this fusion of power and peace, cultivates a deep-rooted sense of tranquility and harmony within your Authentic Self.

True power doesn't come from imposing our beliefs or trying to control outcomes. It stems from a deep well of intrinsic worth and wisdom, a place where words are unnecessary and validation holds no weight. When you remember that you are the bridge to your own happiness and take steps to restore peace in your life, you begin to understand the depth of your power. Your authentic power reveals a truth that goes beyond mere control or domination.

The essence of authentic power is rooted in a profound understanding of your self-worth—a recognition that your identity isn't bound to external validations or belief systems. Your identity is not just your beliefs about the world, politics, religion, yourself, or others.

Think about a time when you've seen someone lash out simply because someone had a differing opinion. It's often because they've intertwined their identity with their beliefs. They feel personally attacked, so they stop responding from a place of passion and start reacting from a place of fear of losing their identity. Their response may seem over the top because it's not just about a disagreement; it's about protecting who they believe they are.

On the other hand, when someone doesn't tie their identity to their beliefs, they create space for growth and connection. This is powerful. They can be vulnerable, lay their cards on the table, and invite others into the conversation without needing to dominate or feel superior. It takes courage to operate from this place of vulnerability, to open oneself up to the perspectives and truths of those around them. This is what it looks like to embody authentic power and peace.

US NOT THEM

In the arena of authentic power, there's no need for a battle of wills or a push for dominance. Instead, there's a meeting of minds, a willingness to listen and understand, and a recognition that every truth is valid in its own right. Leaders who work from power within, rather than power over, are not rigid and unyielding—they are open, receptive, and willing to engage in genuine dialogue. They have moved past independence and now live and lead from a place of interdependence. There is no "them." It is all "us."

Those who try to impose their power on others often come from a place of internal insecurity and a lack of understanding of their own worth. They may see strength in forcing their beliefs onto others, but true strength lies in the ability to meet others halfway and engage in mutual respect and understanding. This shift towards authentic power, rooted in vulnerability and openness, leads us towards true connection and unity in our shared journey.

At the heart of it all, balance reveals itself as the sacred intertwining of power and peace. Your inner strength, that sense of sovereignty and freedom that's always been a part of you, is always there to tap into. It may have gone dormant when you silenced your imagination, but it's always ready to be remembered. When you access that inner power, peace envelops you. There's no rush, no need for external validation. It's about trusting your intuition, your creativity, and embracing the unknown.

If you haven't thought about authentic power in this way before, don't worry—you have the ability to shift your mindset like a superpower. Your imagination holds the key to creating something entirely new, something that hasn't existed before. You imagined yourself into being up to this point, so why couldn't you imagine a new path for yourself?

It's not about seeking external validation but rather realizing your role as the creator of your own journey. It's about being the trailblazer, trusting your instincts and taking bold action. This blend of power and authenticity brings the greatest peace and understanding. It will have you moving in sync with your soul's purpose and tapping into that inner source that has always been within you.

I invite you to tap into your inner wisdom, to embrace the power that resides within your being and discover a profound sense of purpose and understanding—a sacred space where authenticity reigns and the soul finds its true north. The balance we feel through the marriage of power and peace allows us to embrace ideas that spark our inspiration and reflect our Authentic Self. It allows us to access a power that never overpowers or diminishes others. Instead, it creates space for everyone to shine.

PATH TO PROGRESS

Authentic Power and Peace:

- **Affirmation:** *"I balance my inner power and peace, creating harmony in my life."*
- **Soul to Soul Message:** Balance is the marriage of power and peace. Embrace your inner strength without the need for external validation. True power lies in vulnerability and openness, allowing you to connect deeply with others and create genuine harmony.
- **Key Takeaways:** Recognize True Power: Understand that authentic power comes from within, not from imposing beliefs

on others. Embrace Vulnerability: Open yourself to the perspectives of others without feeling threatened. Separate beliefs from identity: Know that your identity is not tied to your beliefs, allowing for more meaningful and respectful conversations. Balance Power and Peace: Find harmony by aligning your inner strength with a sense of tranquility.

☐ **Action Step:** Reflect on a recent situation where you felt the need to assert your beliefs strongly. Consider how you could have approached it differently, using vulnerability and openness instead of dominance. Write down one way you can practice this balanced approach in future interactions. Commit to being mindful of separating your identity from your beliefs, fostering authentic connections.

If you liked this message, you may want to choose your journey to Evolve 1.9 or Emerge 2.9.

Expand Exploration

Reflect on a time when you felt a need to change someone's opinion to validate your own beliefs. How did this impact your sense of inner balance and peace?

Think about a situation where fear prompted you to seek control or dominance. How could you choose differently?

...

3.10
CRAFTING A NEW NARRATIVE

*Write a new ending on each new page of your life,
and let each chapter be a testament to your growth,
courage, and Authentic Self.*

Are you willing to sacrifice your comfort for creativity?

For inspiration? For growth? For expansion?

Your comfort keeps you confined.

You may point to outside sources for your loss of freedom, but the truth is, you often take it from yourself.

Choosing to remain compliant and comfortable prevents you from expanding.

You confine yourself in small quarters, small stories.

The walls of your house continue to press inward on your spirit.

Change. Change the small habits. Change the big ones too.

Your willingness to be grateful for the *new* will signal the Universe to bring you more *new*.

New stories. New adventures. New people. New experiences. New words on the pages of your life.

How can you welcome new and different experiences when you constantly replay the past?

It's time to hit pause. Catch your breath.

B R E A T H E

Breathe in stillness. Breathe in creativity. Breathe in abundance.

Breathe in gratitude. Breathe in freedom. Breathe in balance.

Breathe in authenticity.

Once you have found your center, then proceed with play.

P L A Y

Play with thoughts. Play with choices. Play with joy.

You have outgrown your fears. You have outgrown your smallness.

You laid out your plan long before you remembered to walk it.

L E A D

Lead as your heart would sing. Lead as your light would shine.

Lead as you wish your story to be told.

PATH TO PROGRESS

Crafting Your New Narrative:

- ☐ **Affirmation:** *"I embrace change and creativity, writing a new ending on each page of my life."*
- ☐ **Soul to Soul Message:** Your willingness to step out of your comfort zone and embrace change is the key to expanding your life. By letting go of old stories and habits, you create space for new adventures and experiences.
- ☐ **Key Takeaways:** Embrace Change: Understand that comfort confines you, while change and creativity lead to expansion. Let go of the past: Release the replay of past stories to make room for new possibilities. Breathe and center: Find your balance and authenticity through stillness and gratitude. Approach life with a playful heart, leading with your light and writing your story with joy and intention.
- ☐ **Action Step:** Reflect on areas of your life where you feel confined or stuck. Write down small and big habits you can change to invite new experiences. Practice gratitude daily for the new opportunities that come your way. Spend a few moments each day breathing deeply and centering yourself, then engage in a playful activity that sparks your creativity and joy. Commit to leading your life with authenticity and writing a new, inspiring narrative for yourself.

If you liked this message, you may want to choose your journey to Evolve 1.10 or Emerge 2.10.

Expand Exploration
*What fear is keeping you from writing a
new page to your story?*

*How can you expand your life to try a new activity,
food or adventure?*

• • •

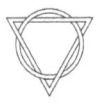

3.11
THE POWER OF LETTING GO
Love others enough to let them live their story.
"To love without condition is the only way to really know love, and the greatest gift we can give another is the freedom to be themselves."
~ Sonia Choquette

Allowing those we care about to follow their own paths means confronting our insecurities and worries. Loving others enough to let them live their story requires stepping back and trusting their ability to navigate life's twists and turns without interference. As Sonia Choquette beautifully states, *To love without condition is the only way to really know love, and the greatest gift we can give another is the freedom to be themselves.*

Recognizing that everyone's journey is unique—filled with lessons, challenges, and growth essential to their personal evolution—is key. By releasing the need to control or direct their narratives, we create space for authentic growth, mutual respect, and a deeper connection rooted in trust and freedom.

THE DEAD END
This lesson became especially clear during a challenging time before my son's high school graduation. We received word that he would not be graduating from PCTI (Passaic County Technical Institute) due to reasons that seemed deeply unjust and unfair. As his mother, I spiraled into a frenzy of emotions. I cried, raged, and fought fiercely—desperate

to make things right. I pushed, prodded, and shouted, demanding justice for my son.

But then, amidst the chaos, I had a moment of clarity. I said something to my sister (ego talking) that I quickly realized my soul didn't agree with: *When will it ever be bad enough that he will learn?*

The minute those words left my mouth, I realized how backwards my ego speaks. My son is powerful, creative, and innovative—he has never fit into the box that our school system, or society for that matter, has created for him. Jordan possesses great perseverance; he doesn't view the end of the road as a dead end but rather as an opportunity for a new turn, much like the swirl of the unalome symbol tattooed on my arm.

As I uttered those words, it was as if I heard a symphony of understanding from the Universe. I knew in that instant this was not how I wanted to live, nor how I wanted my son or anyone else to live. Nothing will ever be so bad that there isn't another choice, another way. I realized that by holding on so tightly to what I believed was 'fair,' I wasn't allowing him to live his own story.

So – I let go.

In the months that followed, I watched as Jordan sat in a seat at our hometown high school for half a year, retaking a class he had already completed. He also had to take gym class again, as required by New Jersey state law for students repeating a year. Jordan showed up, did the work, and never once complained. He even upped his work hours outside of school, tackling life with the quiet strength and resilience that defines him.

One day, during this difficult time, as I stood in the kitchen with tears streaming down my face, Jordan looked at me with calm assurance and said, *It's going to be alright, Mom. I'm going to graduate. It'll still happen, just not the way we thought.* And true to his word, he did exactly that.

His words were a powerful reminder of the lesson I had just learned: things will unfold, but perhaps not in the way we expected. Letting go holds immense power, allowing others to live their own story while we walk beside them, witnessing their journey.

SURRENDER

Our bonds with family, friends, and even ourselves hold powerful healing energy, soothing the scars of both yesterday and today. Loving others enough to give them the freedom to shape their own paths, without our shadows casting doubt, is a profound act of surrender. It requires a deep trust in the wisdom of each person's unique journey. By embracing our true selves, respecting our boundaries, and making decisions based on self-awareness, we build stronger bonds of trust with those around us. Letting go of the urge to shield and guide, we empower others to face their challenges and victories with courage and independence.

We all carry soul contracts, threads of destiny woven with lessons to embrace and opportunities for growth. Just as our soul's journey is personal and intimate, so too are the soul contracts that bind us to our loved ones. Reflecting on shared moments of pain, hope, growth and transformation, we come to understand them not as mere periods of hardship, but as pivotal points of learning and evolution.

I used to believe the saying, *You're only as happy as your happiest child*, but I've since experienced a significant shift. Letting go of this deeply ingrained belief allowed me to understand happiness in a new way.

Now I see that true happiness comes from my own choices and authenticity. Realizing that my inner joy isn't dependent on external validation, I am now on a path of growth and freedom. Understanding the importance of this independent way of living, I can hold space for my loved ones to do the same.

This realization has brought me freedom as I navigate personal growth and support others on their journeys toward happiness and wisdom. By embracing the autonomy of individual happiness and honoring diverse paths, we can become our most authentic selves and thrive in a community of genuine connections.

Each page of our life reveals a new aspect, offering a chance to reshape our story. We consistently stand at the crossroads of endings and new beginnings, linking the past with the present. True liberation comes from releasing our need to control those we hold dear and letting go of the impulse to manage their every step. When we view our regrets not as harsh lessons but as the GPS for growth, we open the door to expansion. By granting our loved ones the freedom to navigate their own paths, we also embark on a parallel journey of rediscovering and accepting ourselves.

Embracing trust, faith and understanding is crucial in relationships. Just as you navigate this book—sometimes reading chapters in order, sometimes skipping around—allow your loved ones the same freedom in their journeys. Trusting them to write their own stories honors both their journey and your interconnectedness.

Each person's story unfolds uniquely, often diverging from your own. By giving them the space to live authentically and embracing their choices, you celebrate self-love and growth. Trusting them with their own narratives enriches your shared existence, weaving it with empathy, understanding, and authenticity.

PATH TO PROGRESS

The Power of Letting Go
Respecting the Individual Journey:

- ☐ **Affirmation:** *"I love others enough to let them live their story."*
- ☐ **Soul to Soul Message:** Embracing love means letting go of the need to control others' journeys. Trust in their ability to navigate life's paths and honor the unique lessons and growth each person must experience.
- ☐ **Key Takeaways:** Embrace Individual Journeys: Recognize that everyone's path is unique and essential for their growth. Release Control: Let go of the need to direct others' lives, creating space for mutual respect and deeper connections. Trust and Freedom: Trust in the wisdom of each person's journey, fostering authentic growth and independence.
- ☐ **Action Step:** Reflect on a situation where you felt the urge to control or direct someone else's journey. Journal about the emotions and fears behind this urge. Write down ways you can practice letting go and trusting their path. Commit to giving them the space to live their story while focusing on your own growth and authenticity.

If you liked this message, you may want to choose your journey to Evolve 1.11 or Emerge 2.11.

Expand Exploration

Where do you need to surrender and allow your loved ones to live their own story?

What fears are holding you back from letting go?

3.12

AUTHENTIC SPLENDOR

Bold. Beautiful. Bountiful.
Live life in the authentic splendor of you.

"We need you to reveal to us what you know, what you have learned, what you have seen and felt. If you are older, chances are strong that you may already possess absolutely everything you need to possess in order to live a more creative life - except the confidence to actually do your work. But we need you to do your work."
~ Elizabeth Gilbert, Big Magic

For longer than I'd like to admit, living boldly, embracing my beauty, and experiencing a bountiful life felt like a distant dream. Authenticity and moments of pure splendor seemed like foreign lands for which I didn't yet have a passport. But I no longer carry regret in this realization. Life's truth unfolds as we move forward, and clarity comes only when we look back. We couldn't be where we are now without having been where we were.

As you learned in previous sections, we all enter this world with specific soul contracts, each yearning to practice, learn and grow. When I found myself feeling unworthy of my beauty, lacking courage or experiencing scarcity, I came to understand it was part of my soul's contract to learn how to embody these very qualities through the experiences I was given. Each challenge and situation is a classroom where we practice and flourish.

Whether it's cultivating compassion, forgiveness, or patience with ourselves or others, we experience the scenarios we need to help us evolve, emerge, and expand into our true selves.

Reflecting from where I stand now, I am reminded of the words of Elizabeth Gilbert, which echo in my mind: *We need you to reveal.* She urges us to share our knowledge, experiences and feelings with the world. Regardless of age, we hold within us everything required for a vibrant life, waiting only for the courage to unleash our creativity and share our stories. This is what it means to expand.

When we practice evolving, we go inward, deciding what beliefs to keep and what to evict. When we practice emerging, we replace limited thoughts with vibrant and authentic truths. And when we practice expanding, we reveal what we know so others can join us on this journey.

In my quest to understand boldness, bountiful living, and authenticity, I discovered that these qualities aren't about grand gestures or outward appearances. They are about embracing who we truly are, celebrating our uniqueness, and relishing the abundance of life's simple joys. Through moments of introspection and growth, I found my way back to my Authentic Self—a place where masks are shed and true essence shines.

This return to my genuine self opened the doors for me to create a space where others could journey alongside me—just as you are doing now—discovering your own path to self-actualization and fulfillment.

I'm grateful this journey is not mine alone. It's an invitation for you to embark on your own path of self-realization, embracing your boldness, beauty and bountiful life to create a space where authenticity lives. This path to self-discovery unfolds through moments that etch themselves firmly into our hearts and minds.

In my younger years, I sought solace in conformity, molding myself to fit the expectations of others. But much changed in my mid-forties as I set my sights on self-discovery and left my desire for conformity behind. My forties became a time of significant shifts and recognition of my Authentic Self, but it didn't end there.

As I entered my 53rd year, I was gently guided by the wisdom of Jacqueline Balloutine, a compassionate and gifted soul. Certified in hypnosis and past-life regression, Jacqueline helped me uncover memories from my past, each revealing a piece of the puzzle to my current existence. One memory stood out vividly: my 12-year-old self, struggling to fit into my own skin, fumbling through uncertainty. It was during this hypnosis session that I came to understand something essential: the triggers and insecurities we face in the present are often rooted in long-forgotten memories from our past.

In fact, a seemingly simple task—like needing to buy a bathing suit for an upcoming retreat—had unexpectedly stirred up deep-seated emotions I didn't even know were still lingering. As we explored these emotions, a memory surfaced, revealing one of the origins of my body insecurities. It centered around a red bathing suit and a family vacation to my grandmother's cottage on the lake.

THE RED SUIT

At twelve years old, I was nearly my current height of 5'7" and well on my way to developing a shapely woman's body. I had no idea what a 'normal' size should be, but hearing the girls snicker and whisper (not so quietly) under their breath made me feel ashamed of my body and created an intense sense of separateness from the other girls my age.

During my hypnosis session, a memory surfaced that revealed one of the origins of my deep insecurities about my body. It centered around a red bathing suit and a family vacation to my grandmother's cottage on the lake. Back then, shopping as a pre-teen was very different from today. There were no stores like Forever 21, Express, or Old Navy. The best a young girl could hope for was to find something in the Women's Department of Alexander's, a store similar to Target or Bosco's. Unfortunately, shopping in the Women's Department meant the style and cut were not made to fit a young girl's body.

As I spun the rack of women's bathing suits, a red suit caught my eye. I had no idea what size I was or whether it would fit, but I was happy when my mother nodded in approval. We took it straight to the

register, skipping the dressing room since we were short on time. It's strange how such vivid memories, forgotten for forty-one years, could resurface so clearly in my hypnosis session, as if no time had passed. Jacqueline fluidly moved me from one scene to the next as if I were watching a movie.

The next vision whisked me to the mirror's reflection, where I saw a distorted image of discomfort and unease as I pulled and tugged at that red suit. Two sizes too small and built for the woman's body I was yet to fully have, I was overwhelmed with embarrassment looking at my reflection.

Although I knew I was safely sitting in Jacqueline's office, I felt the raw emotions of shame and confusion as if I were reliving the experience in real time. Embarrassed and scared, I felt an overwhelming need to dive under the covers and hide, rather than leave the room to join my family at the lake. I looked in the mirror and watched myself yank at the frayed edges of my self-worth. And then the tears began to fall—both in my memory and in the office.

In this realm of hypnotic exploration, I revisited that tender moment, feeling the fabric of the ill-fitting suit chafe against my skin—a physical manifestation of the internal turmoil I struggled to articulate. Each glance mirrored my inner dialogue of inadequacy, amplified by the subtle expressions of discomfort on the faces of the women in my family as I finally joined them at the lake.

My projection became my perception. I judged myself and, in turn, imagined the women in my family were judging me as well, which only reinforced my self-criticism and deepened the feeling of isolation.

Their loving attempts to adjust the poorly fitting garment inadvertently fueled my self-doubt, igniting feelings of shame and unworthiness that lingered for years. The weight of their kindness mirrored my own perceived flaws—a burden I carried long after the swimsuit had been discarded.

THE SIREN'S CALL

Until the session with Jacqueline, my *Little Girl Big* (ego/inner child) believed she was the one at fault. My body. My size. My height. My hips. My stomach. My legs. My breasts. Even though that little girl grew to be 53 years old, she remained the same twelve-year-old hiding within me. Small. Afraid. Unworthy.

She whispered a siren's call of unworthiness: *Stay small, Jennifer. You are too much in that suit. TOO MUCH. Your body does not fit in the world. Stay hidden so you won't need to tug and stretch at the fabric to hide your body. You know how embarrassing it feels to be your Authentic Self. Stay small.* **STAY SMALL.**

At that moment, I could see how the red suit had influenced every situation, conversation, and intimate relationship I'd ever had. With Jacqueline's guidance, I unraveled those tangled threads of self-doubt through introspection, weaving them into acceptance, a deeper compassion and self-understanding for my Authentic Self, who had been waiting for me to remember her.

Leaving the session, I felt a profound sense of clarity. For so long, I believed I was too weak and too small, yet also too big and too much—too unworthy to be seen. But now, I understood the truth: I was never weak or small. My twelve-year-old self had been powerful in protecting me and keeping me safe until I was ready to lift the veil and see with clarity that I was never the wrong fit. I was always perfect. It was the red suit that was not suitable for me.

When I got home, the irony struck me as I received a new bathing suit in the mail. I paused for a moment, absorbing the significance. The incident that had marked the beginning of Little Jen's insecurities had come full circle. But this time, there was no hesitation in trying on the suit. In releasing the grip of self-criticism, I embraced a newfound sense of worth and acceptance, reclaiming the beauty, courage and bountiful essence that had always resided within me.

This realization came just as I was preparing to co-host an international retreat in the coming weeks, where I would need to wear a bathing suit—a task I hadn't faced in years. The initiation into my truest self during my hypnosis session with Jacqueline had been the catalyst. Rather than being challenged by this fear, I befriended it, recognizing it as part of my journey. It no longer held power over me as I embraced this transformative retreat with confidence and self-acceptance.

EMBRACE YOUR JOURNEY

This return to my Authentic Self opened the doors for me to create a space where others could journey alongside me, discovering their own path to self-actualization and fulfillment.

Remember, you were never meant to fit the suit; the suit is meant to fit you. Embrace your story, and recognize that you hold the power to rewrite it to align with your truth. By doing so, you unlock the door to a life of boldness, beauty, and abundance.

As you **evolve**, **emerge**, and **expand**, embrace the authentic splendor of your true self. Let your journey be a testament to the power of self-discovery and transformation. Inspire others to do the same with unwavering boldness and radiant beauty.

This is your journey, your story, your truth—live it fully, proudly, and let your authentic light shine for all to see. You are not just a participant in life but the author of your own narrative. Your unique and powerful path is a beacon of hope and inspiration to those around you.

Along the way, trust the quiet whispers of your intuition. It will guide you when the path feels uncertain, reminding you that you already hold the answers within. Trusting yourself allows you to navigate life's twists with grace and confidence.

Embrace each moment with courage, knowing that every step you take is a testament to your strength and resilience. Your story is woven with threads of triumph, vulnerability and growth. As you continue writing it, may it be filled with chapters of joy, love and profound self-realization.

Live boldly, love deeply, and let your light shine brilliantly. Your life, in all its authenticity, is a gift to the world. Illuminate the path with your brilliance, for you are a living miracle, and your story is a masterpiece in the making.

As you close this book, remember that your journey is ongoing. You have uncovered the depths of your Authentic Self, but this is only the beginning. Every day is an opportunity to evolve, emerge, and expand into the woman you were born to be.

So, continue your journey. Trust yourself, trust your intuition, embrace your worth and live authentically. Your brilliance will transform not only your life but also the lives of those around you.

Thank you for journeying with me. May you continue to rise, shine, and embrace the life that is waiting for you with open arms, an open heart, and the unwavering guidance of your intuition.

PATH TO PROGRESS

Authentic Splendor. Boldness, Beauty, and Abundance:

- ☐ **Affirmation:** *"I live boldly, embrace my beauty, and experience a bountiful life in my authentic splendor."*
- ☐ **Soul to Soul Message:** Embrace your journey and recognize that your challenges are opportunities for growth. Each experience helps you embody boldness, beauty, and abundance, leading you to your true, Authentic Self.
- ☐ **Key Takeaways:** Embrace Your Journey: Understand that every challenge is an opportunity to practice and grow, helping you embody your authentic self. Rewrite our story: Realize that you have the power to change your narrative and evict limiting beliefs, allowing you to live a bold, beautiful, and bountiful life. Live authentically: Celebrate your uniqueness and embrace the simple joys of life, creating a space where authenticity reigns supreme.
- ☐ **Action Step:** Reflect on a moment when you felt limited by others' expectations or your own self-doubt. Write down this experience and identify the limiting beliefs that held you back. Then, rewrite this story from a perspective of boldness, beauty, and abundance. Commit to living this new narrative daily, celebrating your authentic splendor and inspiring others to do the same.

If you liked this message, you may want to choose your journey to Evolve 1.12 or Emerge 2.12.

Expand Exploration

Reflect on a childhood experience that left an emotional scar, shaping a long-held misunderstanding or belief about yourself.

What truths can you share with your younger self now, offering the wisdom and understanding that she lacked during those moments of confusion and self-doubt?

· · ·

Divine Feminine Prayer

Divine Sophia,

Guide us as we embrace the journey of self-discovery, flowing with the wisdom and intuition of the feminine divine. Help us heal our hearts, knowing that in doing so, we heal the world. Let us release old narratives and embrace our true, authentic selves, celebrating our boldness, beauty, and abundance.

Illuminate our paths as we evolve, emerge, and expand. Encourage us to share our stories and knowledge, inspiring others to join us on this journey of transformation. May our light shine brightly, creating ripples of love and healing throughout the world.

As we gather this wisdom and prepare to step boldly into the world, may we carry this strength and insight beyond these pages, continually evolving, emerging, and expanding in the authentic splendor of who we are. Let us live our truth with courage and grace, knowing that our journey is a beacon of hope and inspiration to those around us.

Amen.
And so it is.

Afterword
Your Journey Continues

As you close this book, I want to take a moment to acknowledge the incredible journey you have undertaken. Through the sections of *Evolve, Emerge, and Expand: Return to Your Authentic Self*, you have explored the depths of your being, shedding old beliefs, embracing your true self, and stepping into your power.

This journey is far from over. The path to your Authentic Self is a continuous one, filled with moments of growth, reflection, and transformation. You have now equipped yourself with the tools to navigate this path with confidence and grace.

Next Steps

To continue your journey, I encourage you to:

1. **Journal Regularly:** Reflect on your experiences and insights. Use the prompts provided throughout the book to guide your thoughts.
2. **Practice Meditation:** Stay connected with your heart center through daily meditation. Focus on the themes of love, light, and authenticity.
3. **Take Action:** Identify one action you can take each day to honor your authentic self. This could be setting boundaries, pursuing a passion, or simply taking time for self-care.

Stay Connected

Come join our growing community of like-minded individuals at *https://www.facebook.com/groups/healthywomanmanifest*. Or participate in my upcoming workshops and events designed to support you on your journey. These include:

1. **Online and In-Person Workshops:** Tailored to deepen your understanding and practice of the principles in this book.
2. **One-on-One Coaching and Group Coaching**: Personalized guidance to help you stay aligned with your Authentic Self.
3. **Angel and Affirmation Cards for support**: Specifically, the *Evolve Emerge Expand: Returning to Your Authentic Self* deck, affectionately known as the "Red Dress Deck." These cards are designed to support and remind you of the teachings and insights from this book. Keep them in your pocketbook or bag for daily inspiration.
4. **Annual Women's Retreat:** Come join us every fall for a transformative retreat. It is an amazing space to connect with other powerful, healing women.

A Personal Message

I am deeply grateful for the opportunity to be part of your journey. Your commitment to returning to your Authentic Self is inspiring, and I believe in your power to create a life filled with joy, love, and purpose.

Call to Action

Remember, your light is powerful. By sharing your experiences and stories, you can inspire others to embark on their journey of self-discovery and healing. Together, we can create a ripple effect that transforms the world.

Thank you for allowing me to be part of your journey. I am honored to walk this path with you.

With love and light,

Jennifer

ACKNOWLEDGMENTS

To my mother, who unknowingly set me on a path of leadership and creativity. From as early as I can remember, you were always creating—patterns, clothing, dolls, and costumes. Your endless projects brought joy and excitement to our home, teaching me that we are creators by nature. You showed me the beauty of being in flow, and for that, I am profoundly grateful.

To my father, the man who embraced the role of a loving and supportive father to two daughters. Your unwavering belief in me has been my pillar of strength. You were never afraid to show your emotions, always calling me *"Love"* and expressing your pride in me. Your constant encouragement reinforced the idea that I could achieve anything I set my mind to, and for that, I thank you from the depths of my heart.

To my husband, who has always been my unwavering support. You have stood by me through every wild idea, book, retreat, and class, even when the vision was not clear to you. Your faith in me has been a constant source of strength. Thank you for believing in me, always. Your love and patience have allowed me to pursue my passions without hesitation. You have been my rock, and I am forever grateful for your steadfast presence in my life.

To my firstborn, Jordan Matthew, whose perseverance and joy inspire me daily. Your laughter and humor keep my heart light and my soul smiling. You are a reflection of my own creativity and resilience, encouraging me to continue healing so that you may walk your path with even greater ease. Thank you for showing me that no obstacle is ever too great to overcome.

To Ashlyn Faith, my daughter and best friend, whose fire and tenacity motivate me to be better every day. Raising you has been a journey filled with inspiration. You have shown me the importance of burning down the old to make way for the new. Your willingness to connect with your higher self at such a young age fuels my journey. Thank you for your unwavering belief in me.

To my sister, Diane, who lived authentically even when I struggled with doing so. You were unafraid to be seen as a rebel, teaching me that true rebellion is about embracing one's true self. Your authenticity has been a guiding light for me, showing me what it means to be comfortable in my own skin. Thank you for your fearless example.

To my ancestors, here and crossed over, for the love and guidance flowing through me. Many times, as I sat to write, I felt your presence—guiding, smiling, laughing, and crying with me. Your dreams set in motion the path I walk today. Thank you for the love that continues to guide me.

To the teachers and students who have been a part of my journey. Being a true teacher means being a passionate student. The knowledge and challenges you brought into my life have shaped me into the best version of myself. Your passion for learning and your willingness to challenge me have been invaluable. Thank you for the lessons and the growth.

To my beautiful circle of friends and coaching clients, who have become my family over the years. I admire, learn from, and grow with each of you. Thank you for providing a place where I belong, where I can be my authentic self without trying to fit in. Your acceptance and love have been a source of comfort and strength.

To my mentor, Rob, who has traveled this journey with me for nearly eight years. Thank you for holding space for me without judgment, for allowing me to grow and evolve. Your willingness to give me the freedom to move on or flow in new directions, if I chose, is a testament to your profound support. This permission alone showed me how we have grown equally together. Thank you for your unwavering presence.

For my little soul who knew her power and purpose were too great to be contained in human form, you have always lived in the womb of my heart. Thank you for guiding me and restoring our family with your love and angelic presence.

To you, the reader, you are the center of the wheel. Every person who reads this book and chooses to evolve, emerge, and expand back into their authentic self validates the very essence of why I wrote it. Though these are my words on these pages, it is your intention and your actions that will guide you back to your true nature. Your commitment to your authentic self confirms and validates the very reason these pages have been printed. They are for you, they are for me, they are for all of us as a collective. I honor you as you honor me by choosing this book. It did not find you by accident; your soul called it off the shelf knowing it's time to return to your authentic self.

Finally, to my higher self, my angel team, and all of my guides. This book is created and written with love, woven with strength, loss, gain, light, shadow, pain, and purpose. It is not my energy and thoughts alone but the collective that I tap into—the love and gifts that have been given to me. I give gratitude for the contrast and the truth that have set me on the path for forgiveness and immense gratitude for learning, evolving, emerging, and expanding as I return to my Authentic Self.

∴

ABOUT THE AUTHOR

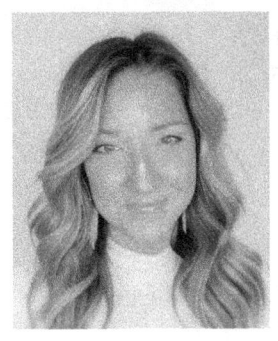

Jennifer is a passionate advocate for women embracing their authentic voice. With a rich background in coaching, keynote speaking, and transformative retreats, she dedicates her life to guiding women back to their true passion and purpose. Her journey of self-discovery and empowerment weaves her experiences into a powerful narrative of wisdom and insight, inspiring women to reclaim their strength and live their most authentic lives.

Jennifer's latest work, "*Evolve, Emerge, Expand: Return to Your Authentic Self,*" exemplifies her commitment to helping women find balance and grace in their lives. Her writing blends professional expertise with relatable, down-to-earth guidance, making it accessible and engaging for women from all walks of life.

Jennifer wrote this book from a place of rebellion against patriarchal expectations. Embracing the rebel archetype within, she chose to write the book in a way that allows women to choose their own paths. Whether they read it from back to front or select one chapter, it is about connecting to their inner desires and needs.

Jennifer is particularly passionate about working with women who are emerging into the second half of their lives with fire, passion, and purpose. Through one-on-one Emergence Coaching and various programs, she helps women embrace this powerful phase of life with confidence and vitality. One of Jennifer's core messages is that every woman has the capacity to shift the direction of her life for herself and future generations. This empowerment comes from recognizing that each woman is the guru of her own life.

Prior to retiring early to commit to supporting women full time, Jennifer was a special education teacher for 27 years. She holds a bachelor's degree in Special Education and a master's degree in Deaf Education. Her focus has always been on clear communication and connecting deeply with individuals on an energetic level, recognizing the unique gifts each person brings to the world.

Jennifer's works, including affirmation decks and oracle cards, reflect her philosophy that life happens for us, not to us, and that empowerment starts from within. She emphasizes the autonomy and sovereignty of a woman's mind, body, and spirit, and the importance of breaking generational patterns from the past.

Nine years ago, Jennifer created the Facebook group *The Miracle Minded Woman* out of a need to find a space where she belonged. When she couldn't find such a space, she created one for others to find her. This group continues to be a haven for women seeking meaningful connections and personal growth.

https://www.facebook.com/groups/healthywomanmanifest.

Jennifer lives in New Jersey but can often be found at her happy place in Cape Cod, Massachusetts, soaking up the sun and the salt air, where she has chosen to host her women's retreat.

Join Jennifer on this journey of self-discovery and empowerment, and let her insights guide you to embrace your authentic self and lead with integrity and passion. For more information, visit *jenkupcho.com*.

Songs for Your Journey: A Musical Compass

As you've journeyed through *Evolve, Emerge, Expand: Return to Your Authentic Self*, these songs have been carefully selected to serve as your musical compass. Each track is paired with a section to deepen your connection to the content, inviting you to reflect, heal, and transform through the power of music. Whether you're revisiting key moments or seeking inspiration, this playlist is here to support your path. You can access the full playlist on Spotify by searching for Evolve. Emerge. Expand. and enjoy this musical guide wherever your journey takes you.

...

YOUR PERSONAL ROADMAP
- **Song:** *I Am Here* by P!nk
- *I Am Here* is an anthem of presence and purpose, fitting for the roadmap that helps you ground yourself in the moment.

PREFACE
- **Song:** *Womankind* by Annie Lenox
- This song celebrates the collective strength and essence of women.

POEMS & PRAYERS
- **Song:** *Women of Hope* by Morley
- *Women of Hope* includes poetry or prayers, as it embodies hope and feminine resilience.

THE COMPASS FOR YOUR JOURNEY
- **Song:** *Soul Sister* by MaMuse
- *Soul Sister* speaks to deep connections and guiding relationships.

EVOLVE

1.1: Embracing Your Worth: Asking for What You Want
- **Song:** *F**kin' Perfect* by P!nk
- This section focuses on embracing your worth, and *F**kin' Perfect* encourages self-acceptance.

1.2: Choose Authenticity Over Approval
- **Song:** *I Am Woman* by Emmy Meli
- This song celebrates authenticity and feminine power, aligning with the message of choosing to be true to yourself rather than seeking approval.

1.3: Transform Through Self-Discovery
- **Song**: *Unwritten* by Natasha Bedingfield
- This song speaks to personal growth and transformation, matching the theme of self-discovery and creating your own path.

1.4: The Magic of Embracing the Unconventional
- **Song:** *Uncharted* by Sara Bareilles
- Embracing unconventional paths mirrors *Uncharted*, a song about stepping into unknown territory.

1.5: Understanding the Non-Linear Path
- **Song:** *Landslide* by Fleetwood Mac
- *Landslide* reflects life's ups and downs, perfectly capturing the essence of the non-linear nature of personal growth.

1.6: Finding Light in the Shadows
- **Song:** *Breaking the Silence* by Marya Stark
- This song connects with overcoming inner darkness and finding your voice.

1.7: Never Abandon Your True Self
- **Song:** *This Is Me* by Keala Settle (from The Greatest Showman)
- *This Is Me* is a powerful anthem of self-acceptance, resonating with staying true to who you are, no matter what.

1.8: Release the Need for Approval
- **Song:** *Stand By You* by Rachel Platten
- *Stand By You* is about standing strong for yourself and others, encouraging you to let go of the need for approval and stand firm in your truth.

1.9: Be the Architect of Your Happiness
- **Song:** *Best Life* by Spencer Ludwig
- This song is an upbeat celebration of choosing to create your own happiness and taking control of your joy.

1.10: Sacrifice Pain to Find Peace
- **Song**: *Breathe Me* by Sia
- *Breathe Me* captures the emotional depth of letting go of pain to find peace, aligning with healing and release.

1.11: Embody Your Unique Essence
- **Song:** *Invincible* by Kelly Clarkson
- *Invincible* is about owning your inner strength and uniqueness, making it a perfect fit for embodying your true self.

1.12: Illuminate Your Inner Light
- **Song:** *Rise Up* by Andra Day
- This song encourages perseverance and shining your light, resonating with letting your inner light illuminate the world.

EMERGE

2.1: Be Your Own Permission Slip
- **Song:** *Unbound* by Rebecca Campbell
- This section encourages stepping into your own power and granting yourself permission to live freely. *Unbound* perfectly matches your limitless potential and living without constraints.

2.2: Go Big: Trust the Process
- **Song:** *A Million Dreams* from The Greatest Showman
- *A Million Dreams* is about having the courage to dream big and trust in the journey, which aligns perfectly with the message of going big and trusting the process.

2.3: Return to Who You Were Created to Be
- **Song:** *I Am Here* by P!nk
- *I Am Here* emphasizes standing in your truth and remembering your purpose; returning to your Authentic Self.

2.4: Be the Host of Your Life
- **Song:** *Shake It Out* by Florence + The Machine
- *Shake It Out* is all about releasing the past and fully stepping into your life, focusing on taking control and hosting your own life.

2.5: Happiness is a State of Being
- **Song:** *Best Life* by Spencer Ludwig
- *Best Life* is an upbeat, positive anthem about choosing happiness and fully living in the moment,

2.6: Embracing Imperfections
- **Song:** *F**kin' Perfect* by P!nk
- This song celebrates imperfections and self-acceptance and embracing all parts of yourself without judgment.

2.7: Life Happens for Us, Not to Us
- **Song:** *Brave* by Sara Bareilles
- *Brave* speaks to taking ownership of your life, stepping up with courage, and understanding that life is happening for your growth reframing how you view life's challenges.

2.8: Embrace Your True Self: Lessons from the Arena
- **Song:** *This Is Me* by Keala Settle (from The Greatest Showman)
- *This Is Me* is all about embracing your true self with boldness and courage and learning from the challenges faced in the arena of life.

2.9: The Transformative Power of Momentum
- **Song**: *Unwritten* by Natasha Bedingfield
- *Unwritten* is about taking steps forward and creating your own future through momentum and transformation.

2.10: The Power of Abundance and Gratitude
- **Song:** *Flowers* by Miley Cyrus
- This song highlights self-love and recognizing abundance in your life; embracing abundance and practicing gratitude.

2.11: Regret as your GPS: Course Correction
- **Song:** *Landslide* by Fleetwood Mac
- *Landslide* reflects themes of introspection, reflection, and personal growth; focusing on turning regret into personal growth.

2.12: The Power of Healing: Emerge as Your Authentic Self
- **Song:** *Stand By You* by Rachel Platten
- This song speaks to support, healing, and standing strong in your truth, which resonates with you emerging as your Authentic, healed Self.

EXPAND
3.1: Choosing Courage Over Comfort
- **Song**: *Brave* by Sara Bareilles
- *Brave* is the perfect anthem for choosing courage, encouraging you to step out of your comfort zone.

3.2: Claiming Your Happiness
- **Song:** *Best Life* by Spencer Ludwig
- This section is all about claiming your happiness, and *Best Life* reflects the joy and empowerment that comes with fully embracing and creating your own happiness.

3.3: The Power of Asking Questions
- **Song:** *The Voice Within* by Christina Aguilera
- *The Voice Within* emphasizes self-reflection and trusting your inner guidance, perfectly aligning with this section's message of the importance of asking questions and seeking answers from within.

3.4: The Power of Belonging
- **Song:** *We Shall Be Known* by MaMuse
- This song is a powerful celebration of community and belonging, matching this section's theme of finding strength and purpose through connection and belonging.

3.5: Navigating the Journey of the Empath
- **Song:** *Never Get Used to This* by Forest Frank
- *Never Get Used to This* reflects the empath's journey of staying open-hearted and appreciating the beauty in life, even amidst the complexity of their own behaviors and emotional challenges.

3.6: The Ripple Effect
- **Song:** *Circle of Women* by Nalini Blossom, Craig Pruess
- *Circle of Women* highlights the interconnectedness and influence we have within communities.

3.7: Subtle Miracles in Everyday Life
- **Song:** *Shake It Out* by Florence + The Machine
- *Shake It Out* speaks to finding light in dark moments and recognizing small, transformative miracles in everyday life.

3.8: The Power of Imagination
- **Song:** *A Million Dreams* from The Greatest Showman
- *A Million Dreams* is a celebration of imagination, creativity, and vision.

3.9: Authentic Power and Peace
- **Song:** *Unconditionally* by Katy Perry
- *Unconditionally* speaks to love, acceptance, and finding peace in being your true self, matching this section's focus on finding authentic power and peace.

3.10: Crafting a New Narrative
- **Song:** *Unwritten* by Natasha Bedingfield
- *Unwritten* is all about creating your own story and rewriting your narrative.

3.11: The Power of Letting Go
- **Song:** *Landslide* by Fleetwood Mac
- *Landslide* is a song of reflection, release, and acceptance of change.

3.12: Authentic Blender: Boldness, Beauty and Abundance
- **Song:** *This One's for the Girls* by Martina McBride
- This song is a celebration of women and the various stages of life, making it a fitting anthem for boldness, beauty, and abundance.

As you listen to these songs, let them be more than just a soundtrack—allow them to be a companion for your ongoing journey. Each melody and lyric is a reminder of the transformation you've embraced, the wisdom you've gained, and the authentic path you now walk. May this musical compass continue to guide you, not just through the pages of this book, but through the many chapters of your life still to unfold. Your journey is unique, and this playlist is here whenever you need to return to your center, reconnect and keep moving forward.